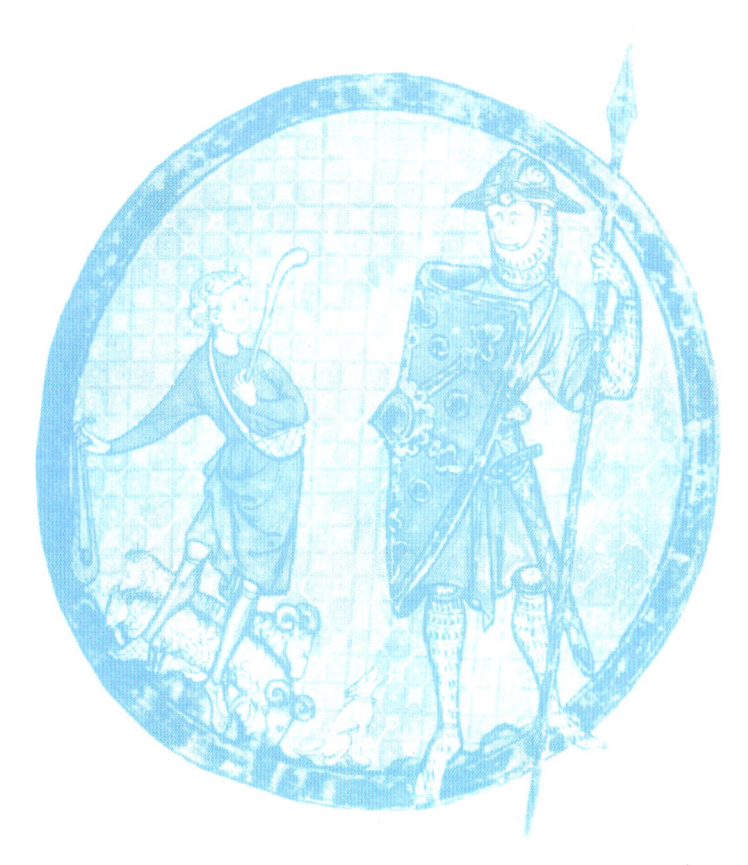

Handbook of Acromegaly

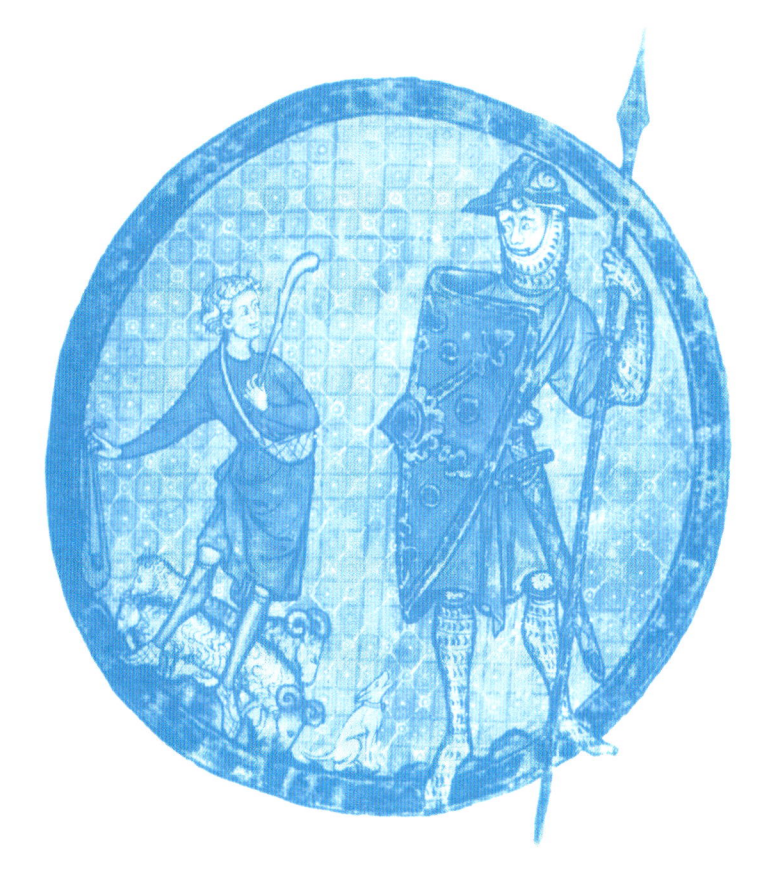

Handbook of Acromegaly
Edited by John Wass

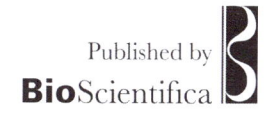

Published by
BioScientifica

Published by
BioScientifica

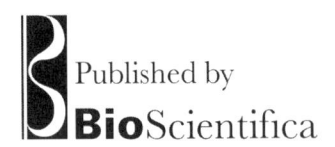

16 The Courtyard, Woodlands, Bradley Stoke, Bristol BS32 4NQ, UK

©2001 BioScientifica Ltd

All rights reserved. No part of this book may be reproduced in any form or by any means without written permission from the publishers.

Disclaimer
The chapters contained in this book have been prepared and written by the named authors. Accordingly, neither BioScientifica Ltd, Novartis nor their officers, employees and agents are responsible for the accuracy or otherwise of any chapters and shall have no liability for any claims, damages or losses however arising from the contents of any chapters or use to which they may be put by any other person.

British Library Cataloguing in Publication Data
A CIP catalogue record for this book is available from the British Library.

ISBN 1 901978 11 7
Cover picture: By permission of The British Library ADD.11639 f523V
Text layout and design by The Designer's Collective
Printed in the UK by Cambrian Printers Ltd, Aberystwyth

PREFACE

The subject of acromegaly, and research into it, engenders intense interest from a wide variety of spheres, medical and other. Happily for our patients, there is good evidence that acromegaly is diagnosed earlier than it was, for example, in the 1930s; early detection prevents the development of some of the irreversible complications of the disease, including osteoarthritis and cardiomyopathy. Nonetheless, we should not be complacent. Particularly in the young, large tumours may sometimes cause the disease before the typical features have developed and we need to be particularly vigilant for these cases, which may go undiagnosed for some years.

It is now an exciting time in scientific terms as well as clinical, because we are gaining insights into the aetiology of the pituitary tumours that cause acromegaly. For the first time since the initial description of the disease, over 100 years ago, we have it within our grasp to control growth hormone (GH) levels and the pituitary tumour itself in the vast majority of patients. This means that, together with the earlier diagnosis alluded to above, we should in future be able to avoid almost completely the serious complications of the disease.

The history of acromegaly and of gigantism is exceptionally interesting. Acromegalic gigantism has been around and described (and often grossly exaggerated) for literally thousands of years. The disease was first described and given its name in the 1880s by Pierre Marie, the French neurologist. In those days, and in the first half of the twentieth century, 30% of patients had visual field defects at presentation. Now this figure is around 10%. This is happy evidence that the disease is being diagnosed earlier, before the tumours are large enough to cause such defects.

Much of the literature on acromegaly has had to contend with historical series that utilise very different GH assays with treatment and follow up extending over many years. Furthermore, the criteria for cure have been evolving constantly, so a study of even the recent literature on acromegaly shows very frequently that different criteria have been used in the measurement of outcome of available treatment modalities. The recent consensus meeting chaired by Andrea Giustina and Shlomo Melmed agreed treatment outcomes in terms of GH and insulin-like growth factor-I (IGF-I) levels and GH responses to glucose. These should be rigorously applied in the scientific and medical communities so that results between different centres can be effectively compared.

Surgical results show considerable variability between experts and those with less experience in the treatment of pituitary tumours. It behoves endocrinologists to refer their patients with functioning pituitary tumours and acromegaly only to those surgeons with a proven track record.

Medical therapy has changed radically in the past few years. It is now possible to gain control in the majority of patients with somatostatin analogues and, for the smaller number of patients resistant to these, pegvisomant, the GH receptor antagonist, appears able to achieve normal IGF-I levels, so that at least in terms of IGF-I we are able to obtain normal levels in nearly 100% of patients. Furthermore, of great interest is the development, currently underway, of new selective somatostatin analogues that act on specific somatostatin receptors.

There are also developments in the field of radiotherapy for acromegaly. In particular, the recent use of stereotactic radiotherapy (radiosurgery) has engendered a great deal of interest and, while we need more long-term data, early results suggest that GH reductions are more rapid with this form of radiotherapy than with other modalities, particularly conventional external beam radiotherapy. For all these reasons, the long-term treatment strategies for acromegalic patients are changing.

It is thus especially timely now to put together a handbook of acromegaly that is easily accessible. The book covers historical and clinical aspects as well as different treatment modalities. It ends with a view of long-term treatment strategies for individual patients with different tumour sizes and with a look forward towards future areas for research.

I am fortunate indeed to have been able to persuade other authors who are all world class experts in their field to contribute to this book. I am very grateful to them for the quality of their contributions as well as the speed with which they have worked. I believe the book will be useful to all who have an interest in acromegaly, including endocrinologists (both trained and in training), neurosurgeons, radiotherapists, physicians and others who see a patient with acromegaly rarely and need some guidance about treatment strategies.

I am particularly grateful to all at BioScientifica, especially Sue Thorn, who has worked with great care and assiduity to ensure the book's rapid and timely emergence. I sincerely hope it is of use to those (including patients) who read it and that it points the way for future research into a condition that has fascinated many and will continue to be of great interest in the future. Undoubtedly, it continues to be a truly exciting time for the advent of the new and more effective treatments for this disease.

John Wass

CONTENTS

Preface		v
The Contributors		ix
Growth Hormone Assays and Units		xiii
Chapter 1	**History of Acromegaly** John A Jane and Edward R Laws	1
Chapter 2	**Clinical Features, Investigation and Complications of Acromegaly** Helen E Turner	17
Chapter 3	**The Aims of Treatment and Definition of Cure of Acromegaly** John Wass	29
Chapter 4	**Surgical Management of Acromegaly** Rudolph Fahlbusch, Michael Buchfelder, Jürgen Kreutzer and Panos Nomikos	39
Chapter 5	**Medical Therapy for Acromegaly** Aart J van der Lely and Steven W J Lamberts	49
Chapter 6	**Radiotherapy for Acromegaly** Paul J Jenkins and P Nicholas Plowman	65
Chapter 7	**Long-Term Treatment Strategies for Acromegaly** John Wass, Steven W J Lamberts and Shlomo Melmed	77
Chapter 8	**Future Areas of Research in Acromegaly** John Wass, Shlomo Melmed and Helen E Turner	85
	Index	91

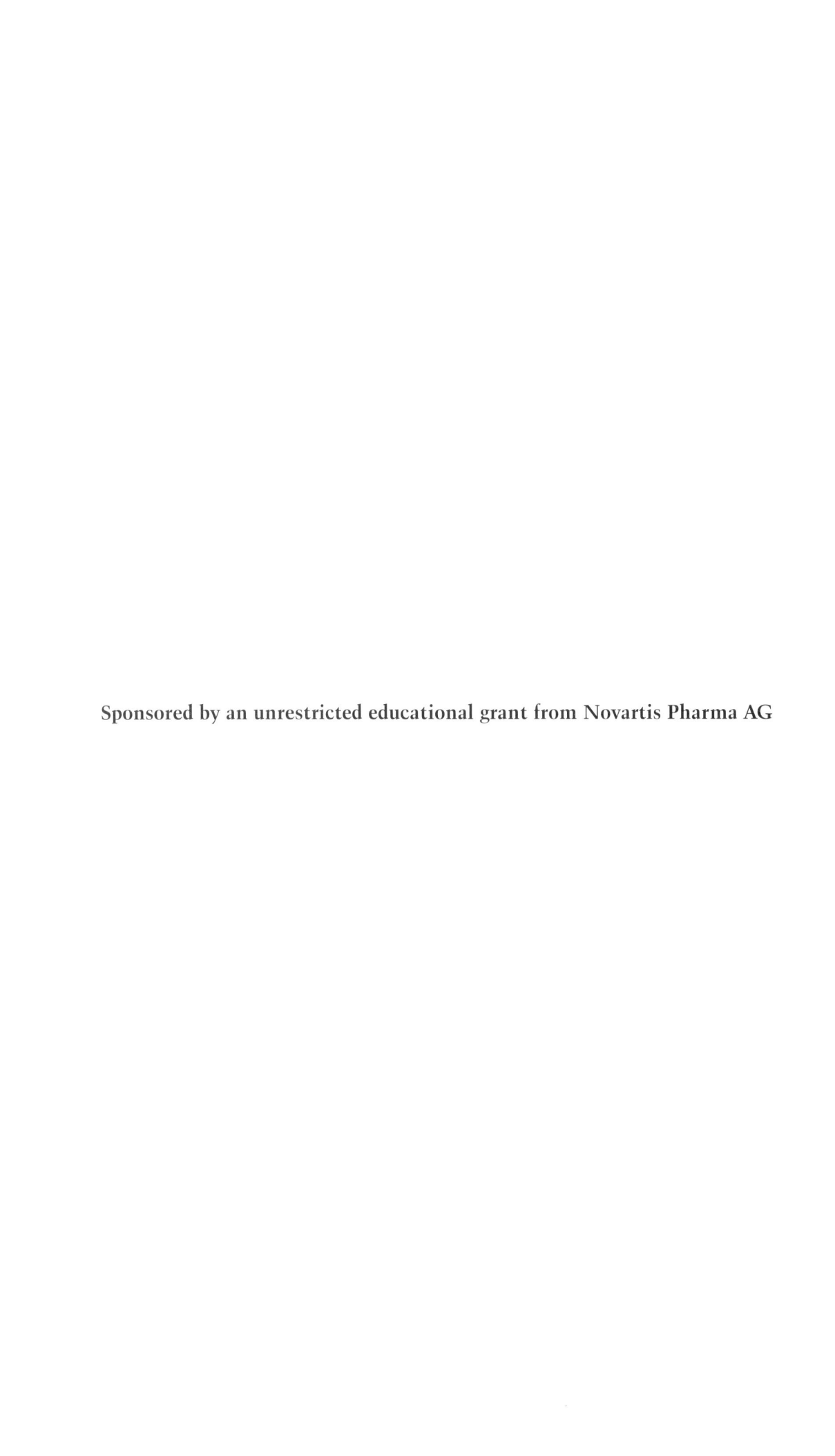

Sponsored by an unrestricted educational grant from Novartis Pharma AG

CONTRIBUTORS

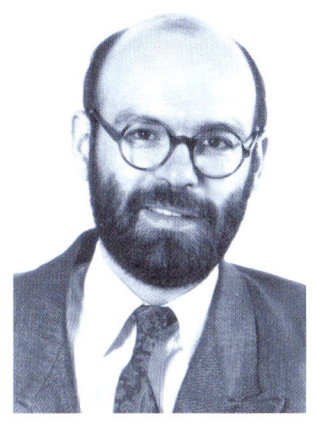

Michael Buchfelder

Prof. Dr med. Michael Buchfelder graduated from the University of Munich Medical School in 1982. His residency training was mainly at the University of Erlangen–Nuremberg, where he also obtained his MD in 1984 for a thesis on *The Effects of Postoperative Radiotherapy of Pituitary Adenoma*. He took part in the training system of the EANS. He became a member of senior staff in 1989, Lecturer in Neurosurgery in 1992 and Associate Professor of Neurosurgery at the University of Erlangen–Nuremberg in 1999. For his lecturership he produced another thesis entitled *Prognostic Factors in Hormone Secreting Pituitary Adenomas*. He is a member of several professional organisations, such as the Endocrine Society, AANS, EANS, CNS and others, and has published some 100 scientific papers in peer-reviewed journals. His main fields of interest include the pathogenesis, diagnosis and treatment of sella region tumours and endocrinological disturbances in other intracranial pathologies, epilepsy surgery, neuronavigation and intraoperative imaging.

Rudolf Fahlbusch

Prof. Dr med. Rudolf Fahlbusch graduated from the University of Munich Medical School. His residency training was at the Neurosurgical Department of the University of Munich and he obtained his MD for a thesis on *Visual Evoked Potentials* at the Neurological Department. He became Lecturer in Neurosurgery in 1977 with another thesis on *Endocrine Functional Disturbances in Cerebral Processes* and Professor of Neurosurgery in 1980. Since 1982 he has been Professor and Chairman of the Department of Neurosurgery at the University of Erlangen–Nuremberg in Erlangen. Significant contributions to neurosurgery include the introduction of neuroendocrinology especially to pituitary surgery, the introduction of approaches to the skull base via the transsphenoidal and the frontobasal approach, basic research in the molecular biology of pituitary adenomas and meningiomas, intraoperative monitoring during microsurgical procedures, especially in the brainstem area, and further developments in computer-assisted surgery, including functional neuronavigation and intraoperative magnetic resonance imaging. He has been honorary and corresponding member of several professional organisations and is a member of the Committe for International Relationship (1998–), EANS, President of the German (2000–2002) and the European Skull Base Society (1999–2001).

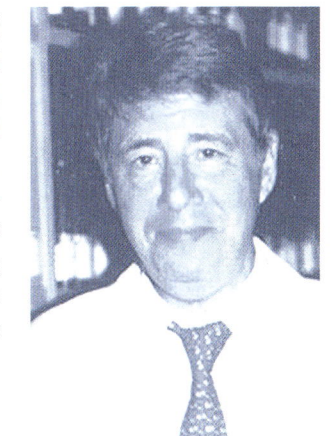

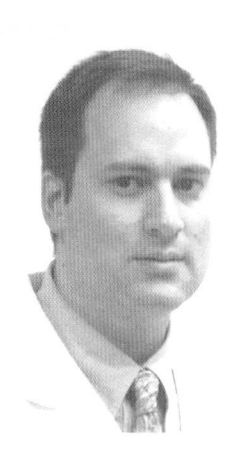

John Jane

Dr John Jane, Jr, is currently a senior resident in Neurosurgery at the University of Virginia. After preparatory school in Charlottesville, Virginia, Dr Jane attended college at the University of Chicago where he studied Art History and graduated with honours. He then returned to Virginia with his wife Robin and attended medical school at the University of Virginia, where he also completed his general surgery internship and began neurosurgical residency in 1997. His wide academic interests range from gene therapy for brain tumours and bone regeneration to paediatric neurosurgery and pituitary disease. After completing residency in 2003, he plans to supplement his training in a paediatric neurosurgery fellowship and then return to Charlottesville to pursue his interests in pituitary surgery.

Paul Jenkins

Having qualified with a degree in Medical Sciences at Cambridge University, Dr Paul Jenkins undertook his clinical training at The Royal London Hospital and graduated in 1988. He has been with the Department of Endocrinology at St Bartholomew's Hospital since 1991, where is currently a Senior Lecturer/ Honorary Consultant. He has a long-standing interest in pituitary disorders, particularly acromegaly, and has been instrumental in establishing the increased prevalence of colorectal neoplasia in this disease. His current major research interests relate to the influence of growth factors in neoplasia, particularly colorectal and breast. He has written numerous peer-reviewed papers and text-book chapters on both clinical and basic aspects of endocrinology.

Jürgen Kreutzer

Dr med. Jürgen Kreutzer graduated from the University of Erlangen–Nuremberg Medical School in 1999. After his internship at the Departments of Anaesthesiology and General Surgery at the University of Erlangen and some scientific and clinical work at the Department of Neurological Surgery in Charlottesville, University of Virginia, USA, he started residency training at the Department of Neurosurgery, University of Erlangen–Nuremberg. He obtained his MD in 2000 for a thesis on *Multiparametric Monitoring of Cerebral Macro- and Microcirculation in Patients with Severe Head Injury*, and became member of the junior staff in 2000. His main fields of interest include the pathogenesis and management of pituitary tumours, tumour biology and tumour cell migration, as well as the pathological implications of altered cerebral autoregulation after head injury.

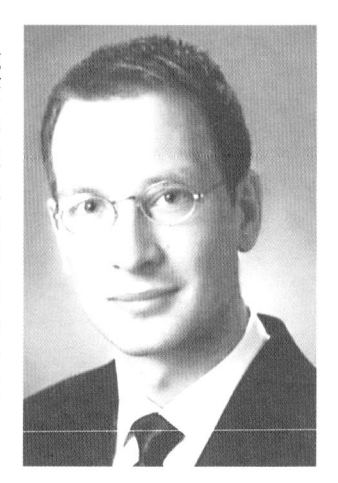

Steven Lamberts

Professor Steven Lamberts is Professor of Medicine at Erasmus University, Rotterdam. He has a special interest in endocrinology, notably pituitary diseases, the endocrinology of ageing, glucocorticoid sensitivity and neuroendocrine tumours. He serves as an editorial board member on a number of endocrine journals.

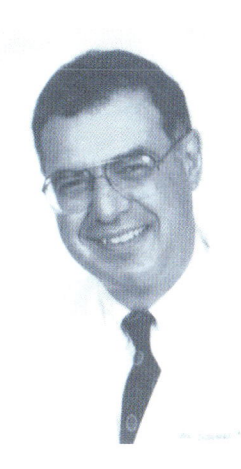

Edward R Laws

Edward R Laws received his bachelor's degree from Princeton University with honours in Economics and Sociology in the Special Program in American Civilization, and then attended the Johns Hopkins University School of Medicine in Baltimore, Maryland, receiving his MD in 1963. He completed his surgical internship and neurosurgical residency at John Hopkins, after which he joined the faculty at the John Hopkins Medical School with a primary appointment in paediatric neurosurgery. In 1972, he joined the staff of the Mayo Clinic in Rochester, Minnesota, where ultimately he became Professor of Neurosurgery and developed major interests in pituitary surgery and epilepsy surgery, along with a continuing interest in the metabolism and pathophysiology of primary brain tumours. In 1987 he became Professor and Chairman of the Department of Neurosurgery at the George Washington University in Washington, DC, and in 1992 joined the faculty of the University of Virginia as Professor of Neurosurgery and Professor of Medicine, establishing a Neuro-Endocrine Center there. During his surgical career he has operated on more than 5000 brain tumours, of which 3600 have been pituitary lesions. Dr Laws has served as President of the Congress of Neurological Surgeons, Editor of *Neurosurgery*, Chairman of the Board of Trustees of the Foundation for International Education in Neurosurgery, Secretary of the World Federation of Neurological Societies, Director of the American Board of Neurological Surgery, President of the American Association of Neurological Surgeons and President of the Pituitary Society. He has authored over 400 scientific papers and book chapters, and with Andrew Kaye is co-editor of the encyclopaedic volume *Brain Tumors*. Currently he is a member of the Executive Committee of the Board of Regents of the American College of Surgeons and is Vice Chair of the Residency Review Committee for Neurosurgery. He remains actively involved in brain tumour and neuroendocrine research.

Shlomo Melmed

Dr Shlomo Melmed received his medical degree from the University of Cape Town School of Medicine in 1970. He is currently Senior Vice-President for Academic Affairs and Associate Dean of the UCLA School of Medicine, and Director of the Research Institute at Cedars-Sinai Medical Center, Los Angeles. He is an elected member of the Association of American Physicians, and the American Society of Clinical Investigation. He is recipient of the Endocrinology Medal of the Royal Society of Medicine and the Pituitary Society's Award for Contributions to Understanding Pituitary Disease, and has been consistently listed in BEST Doctors of America. Dr Melmed's research is devoted to studying endocrine aspects of pituitary neoplasia, molecular pathogenesis and treatment of pituitary tumours, and growth factor regulation of anterior pituitary function. He has pioneered novel medical management strategies for pituitary tumours. Author of over 180 peer-reviewed manuscripts and over 50 book chapters, monographs and reviews he is also Editor of *The Pituitary*, the Neuroendocrine Section Editor for *DeGroot's Textbook of Endocrinology, Williams Textbook of Endocrinology,* and *Harrisons Textbook of Medicine.* He is Editor-in-Chief of *Pituitary* and on the Editorial Board of the *Journal of Clinical Investigation*. He recently completed a 5-year tenure as Editor-in-Chief of *Endocrinology*. He served on the NIH Endocrinology Study Section and has chaired Special Endocrine Study Sections. He is a member of the Council of the Pituitary Society and chairs its Program Committee. He is on the Endocrine Society Council, Program Chair of the International Congress of Endocrinology, 2004, and a member of the Committee for the International Society of Endocrinology.

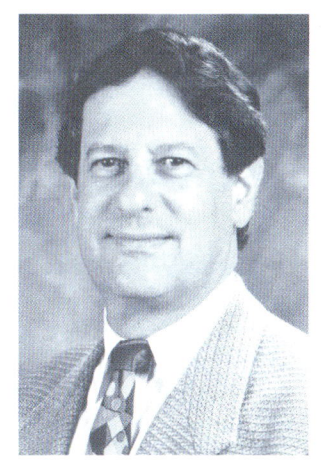

Panos Nomikos

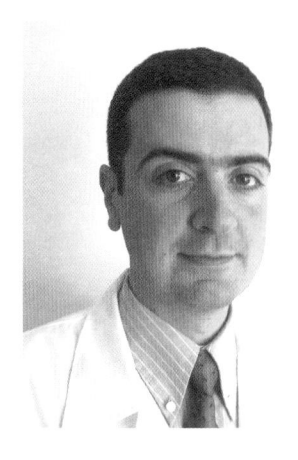

Dr med. Panos Nomikos graduated from the University of Erlangen–Nuremberg Medical School in 1991. His residency training was at the Neurosurgical Department of the University of Erlangen–Nuremberg. He obtained his MD in 1993 for a thesis on *Dopamine D1 Receptors in Cerebral Meningiomas* and became member of the senior staff in 2000. His main fields of interest include the pathogenesis and the management of pituitary tumours as well as skull base surgery.

Helen Turner

Helen Turner graduated in Medicine from Cambridge University and St Bartholomew's Hospital Medical College. She has specialised in endocrinology, and was recently appointed as a Consultant Physician in Oxford. Her research interest is tumours of the pituitary gland and includes clinical studies in acromegaly and laboratory investigation into the role of angiogenesis in pituitary tumours.

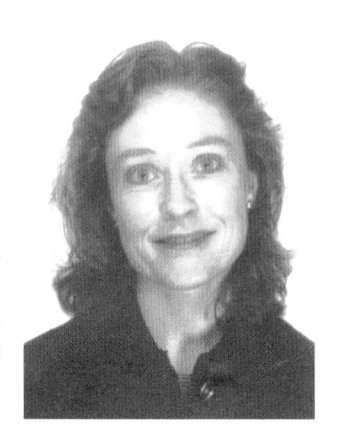

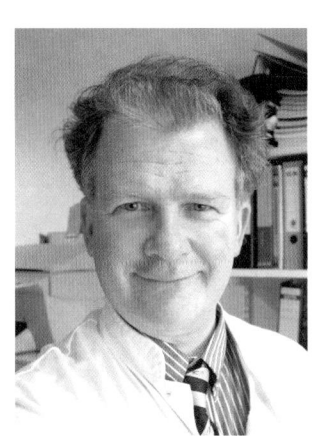

Aart Jan van der Lely

Aart Jan van der Lely is Head of the Division of Endocrinology at Erasmus University Rotterdam. He has a special interest in endocrinology, especially pituitary disorders and endocrine control of metabolism.

John Wass

Professor John A H Wass is Head of the Endocrine Department in the Oxford Centre for Diabetes, Endocrinology and Metabolism at the University of Oxford, UK. His work centres around the treatment of pituitary tumours, in particular acromegaly and the study of growth and growth factors. His research interests also include the genetics of osteoporosis and autoimmune thyroid disease and the development of new pharmacological therapies for pituitary tumours. Before coming to Oxford in early 1995, Professor Wass was a consultant at St Bartholomew's and Professor of Clinical Endocrinology (University of London). John Wass was the Editor of *Clinical Endocrinology* for 4 years until 1995. He is the Vice President of The European Federation of Endocrine Societies and Chairman of the Clinical Committee of the Society for Endocrinology. He was Linacre Fellow at the Royal College of Physicians until 1999. He was President of the Endocrine Section of the Royal Society of Medicine until 1998. He is well-known internationally and has published over 200 papers and 30 book chapters, and edited books including *Clinical Endocrine Oncology*, 1997, and the *Oxford Textbook of Endocrinology*.

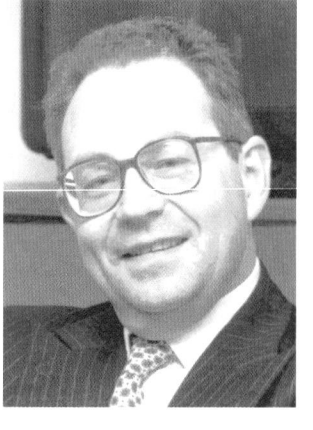

GROWTH HORMONE ASSAY AND UNITS

Readers of this handbook may find it useful to have a short summary of the development of growth hormone (GH) assays to explain the variety of units and conversion factors found in the literature.

The first International Standard (IS) for GH was established for bovine GH in 1955. This was a bioassay and a potency of 1 IU/mg was assigned. It was quickly demonstrated that human GH is species specific and that animal GH is ineffective in humans.

The development of immunoassays during the 1960s led to the first standard for human GH in 1969. The mean of many estimates in four laboratories was used to calibrate the GH content. At that time it was not possible to define GH content in micrograms, so a decision was taken to define content as 2 IU/mg. However, it should be recognised that this was an arbitrary decision.

The first IS for human GH was established in 1982 using the results of a collaborative study that combined bioassays and immunoassays. The best estimate led to a declared content of 4.4 IU/ampoule, which represents approximately 2.5 IU/mg.

By the end of the 1980s this standard was no longer acceptable because of the move to use somatrophin (rDNA-derived GH). In addition, more accurate assays were now available including physicochemical assays. The potency figures derived by the manufacturers of GH ranged from 2.6 to 3.3 IU/mg and a figure of 3 IU/mg was finally settled upon. It is likely that this factor will continue to be used when the next IS is established.

The above summary shows that there is no single 'accurate' conversion factor between IU and micrograms. In this book, each author has been permitted to choose whether to specify GH levels in mU/l or μg/l. Whichever is selected, the other unit is given in brackets, using a conversion factor of 2:1 unless specified otherwise by the author. This conversion factor is used herein as it is the one used by most clinical endocrinologists, but it is every bit as arbitrary as the factors discussed above.

FURTHER READING

Bristow A 1999 International Standards for Growth Hormone. *Hormone Research* **51**(Suppl.) 7–12.

1

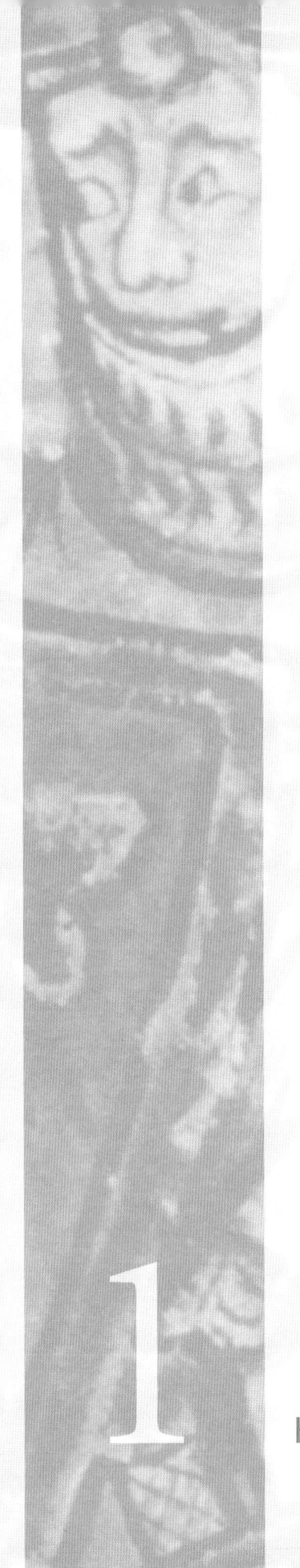

HISTORY OF ACROMEGALY

1 HISTORY OF ACROMEGALY

John A Jane Jr and Edward R Laws Jr Department of Neurosurgery, University of Virginia Health System, Charlottesville, Virginia, USA

INTRODUCTION

Societal interest in giants is nearly ubiquitous across cultures and time. This interest was not lost on the scientific community, who, after the initial description of acromegaly in the late 19th century, focused on discerning its pathogenesis. These efforts led to an appreciation of the endocrine system and, particularly, the hypothalamic–pituitary axis. As this understanding improved, clinicians sought novel therapies and began to assess outcome critically. Although the historical perspectives discussed herein foreshadow the material in the forthcoming chapters, an effort is made to end the discussion prior to the advent of our current therapies.

HISTORY OF GIANTS

Legendary giants

Giant mythology is common to cultures throughout the world (Table 1.1). Judaeo-Christian tradition contains several references to giants. The most famous biblical giant, Goliath (Fig. 1.1), champion of the Philistines, is said to have stood just over six cubits, or 9 feet (2.5 m; 1 Samuel 17:4). In Deuteronomy, King Og of Bashan's bed measured nine cubits, or about 13.5 feet (4 m). Giants played a more central role in ancient Greek mythology. The Greek poet Hesiod fabled that giants were the sons of Gaea (earth) and Uranus (heaven). In a struggle against the Olympians (Gigantomachy), the giants were slain

Table 1.1 The history of giants.

HISTORY OF GIANTS	
Legendary giants	**Historical giants**
Biblical	*Giants of Kings*
Goliath, >9 feet (>2.7 m; Fig. 1.1)	Charles I of England:
King Og, who required a bed measuring over 13.5 feet (4 m)	• William Evans (7 feet 6 inches (2.29 m)), porter
Ancient Greece	• Antony Payne (7 feet 4 inches (2.24 m)), the Cornish giant, bodyguard
Titans	Frederick William of Prussia:
Antaeus	• Potsdam giants
Orion	
Cyclops (Polyphemus)	*Touring Giants of the 18th and 19th centuries*
Norse	Maximilian Christopher Miller (German giant, 7 feet 8 inches (2.3 m))
Aurgelmir	Charles Byrne (Irish giant, 7 feet 6.38 inches (2.30 m); Fig. 1.2)
British Isles	Patrick O'Brien (Irish giant, 8 feet 1 inch (2.46 m))
Corineus, the Trojan, versus Gogmagog, the Cornish giant	Chang Nu Sing (Chinese giant, 8 feet 2 two inches (2.49 m); Fig. 1.3)
Fionn mac Cumhaill	Victorian marriage of 1880 between Anna Swan (Nova Scotia giant, 7 feet 11 inches (2.41 m)) and Captain Bates (7 feet 9 inches (2.36 m))
Far East	
Tibetan Yeti, or Abominable Snowman	*Tallest human on record*
North America	Robert Pershing Wadlow, the Alton Giant (8 feet 11 inches (2.72 m); Fig. 1.4)
Sasquatch, or Bigfoot	
Pecos Bill	
Paul Bunyan	

3

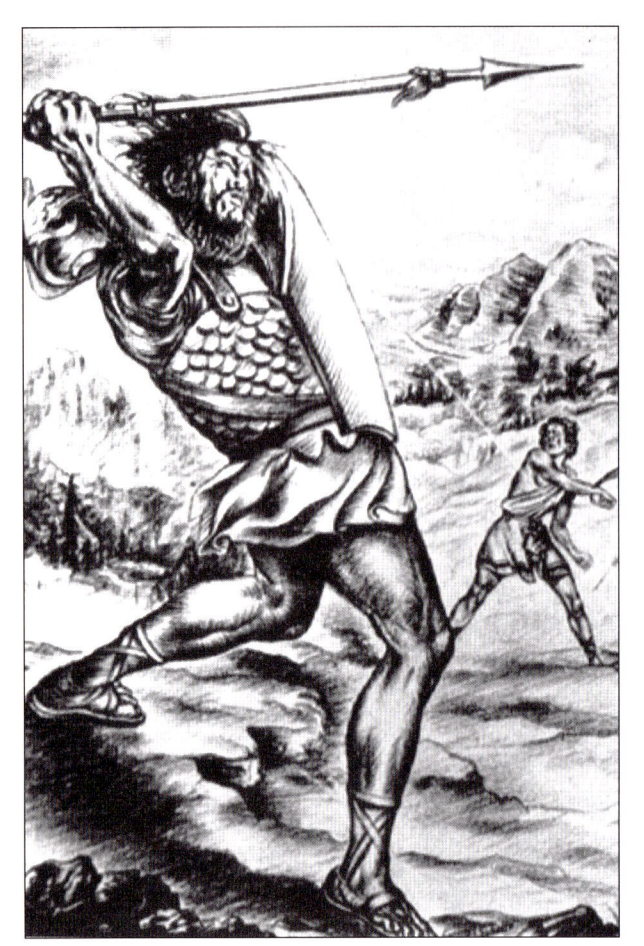

Figure 1.1 David and Goliath, by Gordon Schulte. (Reproduced from Jae Lee (1970), courtesy of AS Barnes and Co.)

and buried under the earth, forming mountains. Other famous giants of Greek mythology include the Titans, Antaeus, Orion and the cyclops Polyphemus, all of whom were offspring of the gods. Giants were central to Norse mythology as well. Aurgelmir, known as the first being, was the father of all giants. After his defeat at the hands of several Norse gods, his body was used to fashion the earth.

Medieval British tradition recounts that the Trojans Corineus and Brutus defeated Gogmagog, a giant who inhabited Cornwall, and subsequently founded Britain. The Giant's Causeway, a massive rock formation in Northern Ireland, is fabled to have been constructed by the Irish giant, Fionn mac Cumhaill.

Far Eastern cultures also provide tales of giants. The Tibetan Yeti, also known as the Abominable Snowman, was a mythical giant thought to inhabit the snowline of the Himalayas. An equivalent being is represented in North American Indian culture as Sasquatch (from the American Indian Salish word 'se'sxac' meaning 'wild men'). Sasquatch, known in American folklore as Bigfoot, was believed to roam the woods of the northwestern United States and western Canada. Legends of these beings persist and alleged sightings continue to be reported.

Giants have also been glorified in North American popular culture. Pecos Bill, the fictitious character popularised by Edward O'Reilly in *The Century Magazine*, was the idealised giant cowboy of the Pecos River region of Texas. Similar oral traditions arose around the heroic giant lumberjack, Paul Bunyan, who is said to have created Puget Sound and the Grand Canyon. James MacGillivray first wrote accounts of his adventures in 1910.

Historical giants

The tales of these fictitious giants were likely spawned from experiences with actual individuals who attained great physical stature during their lives. References abound that affirm the great physical stature of individuals who lived in the latter half of the last millennium. In the 17th century Charles I of England's porter, William Evans (7 feet 6 inches (2.29 m), and his body guard, the Cornish Giant Antony Payne (7 feet 4 inches (2.24 m)), were renowned for their height and physical prowess. Other kings also availed themselves of the service of giants. When enthroned in 1713, Frederick William of Prussia recruited a private militia composed solely of giants (Potsdam Giants).

In the 18th and 19th centuries giants were the subject of great public interest and they toured Europe exchanging personal appearances for money. Some of the notable touring giants were Maximilian Christopher Miller (German giant, 7 feet 8 inches (2.3 m)), Charles Byrne (Irish giant, 7 feet 6.38 inches (2.30 m); *Fig. 1.2*), Patrick O'Brien (Irish giant, 8 feet 1 inch (2.46 m)), and Chang Nu Sing (Chinese giant, 8 feet 2 two inches (2.49 m); *Fig. 1.3*). The 1880 marriage of two giants, Anna Swan (Nova Scotia giant, 7 feet 11 inches (2.41 m)) and Captain Bates (7 feet 9 inches (2.36 m)), was dubbed the Victorian Marriage and provoked significant public interest. The most celebrated giant of the 20th century was Robert Pershing Wadlow (1918–1940), the Alton Giant who stood 8 feet 11 inches (2.72 m) tall and remains the tallest man ever recorded (*Fig. 1.4*).

The public's interest in giants was taken up by the medical profession. At the time of his death in 1783, Charles Byrne's skeleton was acquired for display in the Hunterian Museum of the Royal College of

HISTORY OF ACROMEGALY

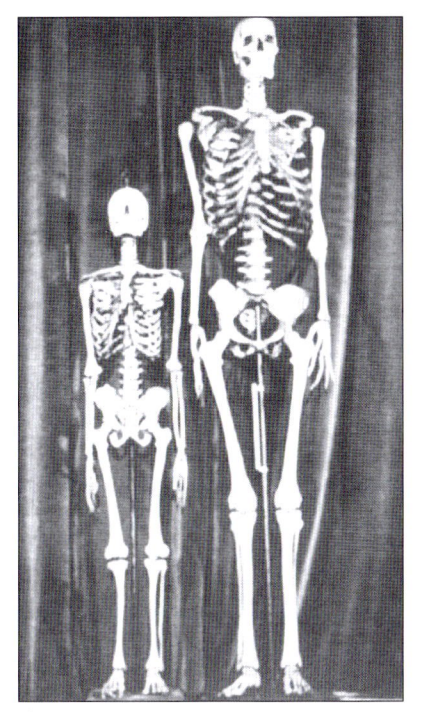

Figure 1.2 Skeleton of Charles Byrne, 1761–1783 (right) in the Hunterian Museum. (reproduced with permission of the Hunterian Museum)

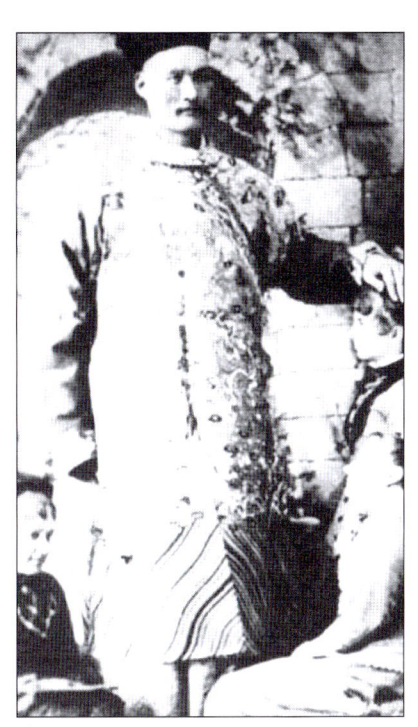

Figure 1.3 Chang Nu Sing, 1841–1893, the Chinese giant; original photograph by Bernard Kobel. (Reproduced from Jae Lee (1970), courtesy of AS Barnes and Co.)

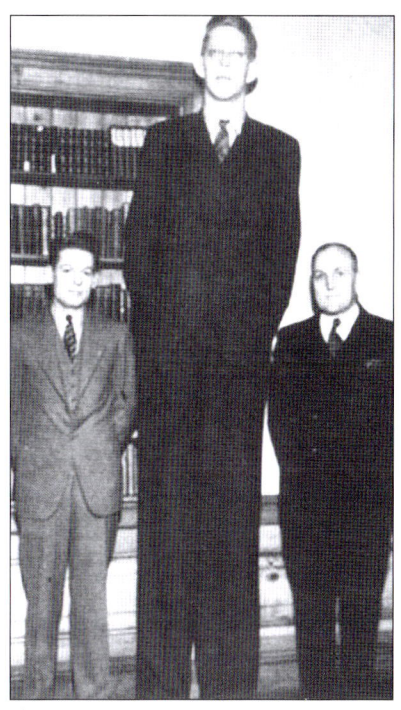

Figure 1.4 Robert Pershing Wadlow, 1918–1940; original photograph by the Alton Evening Telegraph. (Reproduced from Jae Lee (1970), courtesy of AS Barnes and Co.)

Surgeons, London. Later, at the behest of Harvey Cushing, who had great personal interest in giants, Byrne's skull was opened and an eroded sella turcica was discovered. Although Byrne certainly suffered from an adenoma that secreted growth hormone (GH), there is little question that many other giants in history suffered from the spectrum of diseases known to be associated with excess growth. Physicians over the past two centuries have striven to define the distinguishing clinical features and pathoaetiology of acromegaly.

HISTORICAL DESCRIPTIONS OF ACROMEGALY

In 1864, Andrea Verga provided one of the earliest descriptions of the clinical features associated with acromegaly (*Table 1.2*). He termed the syndrome 'prosopectasia' from the Greek 'prosopon' (meaning face) and 'ektasis' (meaning enlargement; *Fig. 1.5*). At autopsy, he noted that the patient had a pituitary tumour, but believed that the syndrome and the tumour had been caused by her early loss of menses.

In 1881 Vincenzo Brigidi reported on the autopsy findings of an Italian actor, Ghirlenzoni, who also had a clinical description consistent with acromegaly. His pituitary, along with other hollow viscera, was noted to be enlarged and hypertrophic. Misinterpreting the

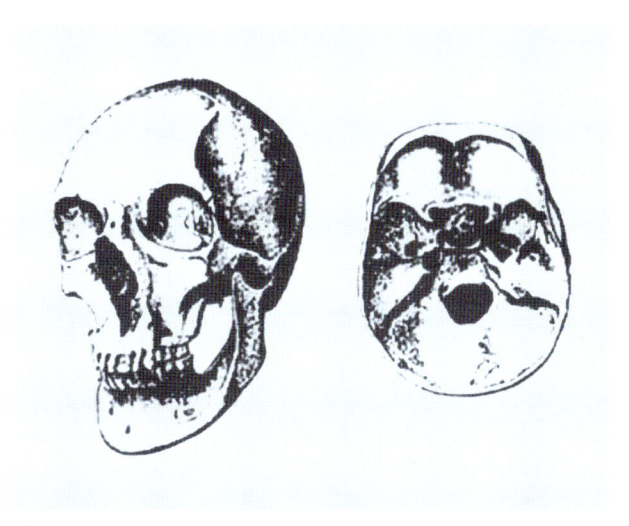

Figure 1.5 Illustration from Andrea Verga's 1864 description of prosopectasia.

HISTORICAL DEVELOPMENTS IN THE STUDY OF ACROMEGALY	
Clinical description	
1864	Andrea Verga, 'prosopectasia'
1886	Pierre Marie, 'acromegaly'
1892	Massalongo, acromegaly and gigantism part of same pathological process
Pituitary source for acromegaly	
2nd C	Galen of Pergamum, phlegm
1892	Massalongo, pituitary hyperfunctioning?
1889	von Mering and Minkowski, produce diabetes by pancreatectomy
1900	Benda, eosinophilic cells in pituitary masses as evidence of hyperfunctioning
1902	Bayliss and Starling, endocrine system
1912	Cushing, *The Pituitary Body and its Disorders*
1921	Evans and Long, experimental acromegaly in rats by injection of pituitary extracts
Growth hormone action and somatomedins	
1927	Smith, experimental hypophysectomy
1939	Freud *et al.*, GH increases tibial epiphyseal width
1953	Ellis *et al.*, growth effects by sulphation of cartilage
1957	Salmon and Daughaday, GH actions mediated by 'sulphation factor'
1963	Glick, Hunter, Utiger, Roth, bioassay for GH available
1972	Daughaday *et al.*, propose name 'somatomedin'
Regulation of growth hormone secretion	
1960	Reichlin, abnormal growth in rats after hypothalamic lesion
1963	Roth *et al.*, pituitary stalk section abolishes hypoglycaemic-induced growth-hormone secretion
1964	Deuben and Meites, hypothalamic extracts stimulate GH secretion, ?GH-releasing factor
1968	Krulich *et al.*, hypothalamic extracts inhibit GH secretion, ?somatotrophin release-inhibiting factor (SRIF)
1973	Ling *et al.*, SRIF (somatostatin) isolated and sequenced

▲ **Table 1.2** Historical developments in the study of acromegaly.

tumour for mere hypertrophy, he considered the aetiology to be a primary disease of the bone. In 1886 the French neurologist Pierre Marie coined the term 'acromegaly' (from the Greek 'akron' meaning extremity and 'megas' meaning great) in his medical description of two patients he had treated at the Salpêtrière Hospital of Paris (Marie 1886). Within the next decade, several authors had correlated gigantism and acromegaly and considered them to be part of the same disease, gigantism being acromegaly of the young (Brissaud and Meige 1895, Massalongo 1892). Although Marie later reported that an enlarged pituitary was universally evident at the autopsy of individuals with acromegaly, he remained uncertain whether it was simply part of the general process of organomegaly seen in the disease (Marie and Marinesco 1891).

■ THE ROLE OF THE PITUITARY

Much of the confusion surrounding the role of the pituitary in disease stemmed from both a misunderstanding of the physiological role of the pituitary in human physiology and a lack of appreciation as to the existence of the endocrine system. Galen of Pergamum, the 2nd century Greek physician, proposed that the pituitary secreted one of the four bodily humours, phlegm, a mucus-like substance that lubricated the nose. This concept remained largely unchallenged until the 19th century.

By 1877 neurones were known to be capable of secreting substances into the blood stream (Du Bois Reymond 1877). Expanding on the work by Claude Bernard on the role of the pancreas in human physiology (Anonymous 1985), in 1889 von Mering and Minkowski published a pivotal work, one now considered the foundation of endocrinology. Noting that diabetes resulted from pancreatectomy, but did not occur following simple pancreatic duct ligation, they proposed that the pancreas acted as a 'ductless gland'. Shortly thereafter, Bayliss and Starling (1902) followed these findings with a report that clarified the concept of the endocrine system. These works provided the basis for speculation on the role of the pituitary in normal physiology and disease.

In 1892 Massalongo suggested that the cause of acromegaly was pituitary hyperfunction. In 1900 Benda proposed that the eosinophilic cells found in pituitary masses were the source of this hyperfunction. Cushing reported in 1909 that the clinical symptoms of acromegaly remitted after partial hypophysectomy, which further supported the pituitary as the source of acromegaly (Cushing 1909a, 1909c). After 3 years Cushing expounded on the central role of the pituitary in the human endocrine system and postulated that certain diseases could be explained by either pituitary hypo- or hyperfunction (Cushing 1912). The pituitary source of acromegaly was confirmed through experiments by Evans and Long (1921), who reproduced acromegaly in rats by intraperitoneal injection of anterior pituitary extracts.

SEARCH FOR PATHOAETIOLOGY

Studies on growth hormone action and discovery of the somatomedins

Such pituitary extracts continued to be used in experiments to study the physiological role of GH. In 1939 Freud et al. demonstrated that GH increased tibial epiphyseal width, and in 1947 Kinsell et al. used this method as a bioassay and confirmed that serum from acromegalic patients could similarly increase the epiphyseal width. By 1953, this growth-promoting effect was shown to relate to sulphate incorporation into cartilage (Ellis et al. 1953). It was not until 1957, however, that Raben was able to isolate human GH. By 1963 a suitable radioimmunoassay became available and GH levels were shown to be elevated in acromegalic patients (Hunter and Greenwood 1962, Utiger et al. 1962, Glick et al. 1963).

Investigations into the physiological action of GH led to the discovery of the somatomedins. Studies were facilitated by Smith's 1927 description of a rat model of hypophysectomy, which allowed researchers to study the actions of injected pituitary extracts in the absence of pituitary influence. In the mid-1950s GH was shown to restore the ability of hypophysectomised rats to incorporate labelled sulphate into cartilage (Murphy et al. 1956). At the same time, however, in vitro experiments revealed that while serum from rats could provoke incorporation of labelled sulphate in cartilage from hypophysectomised rats, GH alone could not (Salmon and Daughaday 1957). These observations led to the concept that GH action was mediated by what was initially termed a 'sulphation factor' (Salmon and Daughaday 1957). Using these in vitro bioassays, sera from acromegalic patients were shown to contain elevated levels of this sulphation factor (Daughaday et al. 1959). By 1972, it was understood that this mediator influenced more than cartilage growth and the broader term somatomedin was proposed (Daughaday et al. 1972). Within 5 years a radioimmunoassay for somatomedin-C (insulin-like growth factor-I) became available (Furlanetto et al. 1977).

Studies on the regulation of growth hormone secretion

With GH identified, other researchers investigated the role of the hypothalamus in regulating GH secretion. In 1960 Reichlin demonstrated abnormal development in rats after hypothalamic lesions and proposed that the hypothalamus probably regulated GH secretion. A further 3 years on, Roth et al. (1963) affirmed this regulatory role by sectioning the pituitary stalk and abolishing hypoglycaemic-induced GH secretion. Central to their observation was their development of a suitable bioassay that could accurately measure GH levels. In the following year this allowed Deuben and Meites (1964) to show that hypothalamic extracts could cause GH release. The establishment of a circadian variation of GH levels also lent credence to the existence of a hypothalamic-releasing factor (Quabbe et al. 1966, Takahashi et al. 1968).

The search for this GH-releasing factor led to the discovery of somatostatin. Krulich et al. reported in 1968 that, although some hypothalamic extracts caused GH secretion, others inhibited its release. Within 5 years the somatotrophin release-inhibiting factor (SRIF), also named somatostatin, had been isolated and sequenced (Brazeau et al. 1973, Ling et al. 1973). As of 1973, the chemistry of GH (Niall et al. 1973) and somatostatin (Brazeau et al. 1973) had been described, but the chemical structure of GH-releasing hormone (GHRH) would not be known for another decade (Guillemin et al. 1982, Rivier et al. 1982).

HISTORICAL TREATMENTS

External radiation therapy

Conventional radiation therapy was first described in acromegalic patients by Béclère in 1909 and independently by Gramegna of Venice in the same year. Radiation therapy remained the first-line treatment at most centres, because of its apparent low morbidity and efficacy in relieving the outward signs of the disease (Table 1.3). As a suitable radioimmunoassay for GH was not available, there were few objective measures of efficacy. Outcomes could only be described in terms of reversing preoperative visual field deficits, control of headaches and remission of signs and symptoms of excess GH. Early studies reported that radiation therapy could improve preoperative visual field deficits in 40–85% of patients (Sheline et al. 1961, Pistenma et al. 1976). Symptoms of GH hypersecretion could be controlled in 80–90% of cases after a considerable lag time, provided that doses of at least 40 Gy were employed (Sheline et al. 1961, Lawrence et al. 1962, Kramer 1973, Pistenma et al. 1976).

The introduction of a reliable GH assay in 1963 caused many investigators to reassess the efficacy of conventional radiation therapy. Satisfactory results were considered to be GH levels below 10 or 5 µg/l (20 or 10 mU/l). The initial reappraisals of conventional radiation therapy indicated that, although it could improve acromegalic symptoms, it was rarely effective at reducing GH levels to normal (Beck et al.

Table 1.3 History of treatment of acromegaly.

HISTORY OF TREATMENT OF ACROMEGALY	
1892	F T Paul, first transcranial surgery for acromegaly, no tumour removed
1906	Sir Victor Horsley, first successful transcranial surgery for pituitary lesions
1907	Herman Schloffer, first transsphenoidal operation for sellar lesion
1908	Hochenegg, first transsphenoidal operation for acromegaly
1909	Harvey Cushing, first transsphenoidal operation for acromegaly, and popularises the approach in the USA
1909	Béclère, conventional radiation therapy for acromegaly
1921	Oskar Hirsch, proposes interstitial radiation therapy for pituitary tumours
1928	Cushing abandons the transsphenoidal in favour of the transcranial approach
1936	Oestrogen therapy relieves acromegalic symptoms
1952 and 1953	Huggins and Bergenstal, adrenalectomy improves outcome in patients with breast and prostate cancer; Poulsen, improvement in diabetic retinopathy after apoplexy; impetus to refine methods of hypophysectomy
1955	Forrest and Peebles-Brown, interstitial radiation for cancer
1959	Fraser, interstitial radiation for diabetic retinopathy
1961	Joplin, interstitial radiation for acromegaly
1963	Glick, Hunter, Utiger, Roth, bioassay for GH causes reassessment of contemporary therapies
1964	Rand et al., stereotactic cryohypophysectomy
1964	Ray and Horwith, transcranial surgery for sellar lesions safe
Late 1960s	Hardy, selective adenomectomy
1967	Zervas and Gordy, stereotactic radiofrequency ablation for acromegaly
1969	Cryer and Daughaday, GH secretion in acromegaly, not autonomous of hypothalamic influence
1960s to early 1970s	Medroxyprogesterone, oestrogen, phentolamine, chlorpromazine, serotonin antagonists tested for efficacy
1972	Liuzzi et al., l-dopa paradoxically reduces GH levels in acromegalic patients
1973	Hall et al., somatostatin infusion reduces GH levels in acromegalic patients
1975	Thorner et al., dopamine agonist, bromocriptine, effectively reduces GH levels

1965, Roth et al. 1967). Radiation therapy evolved and doses were adjusted. The introduction of megavoltage radiation and proton beam therapy improved efficacy in reducing GH levels (Roth et al. 1970, Lawrence et al. 1971). Heavy particle and proton beam radiation were considered the most effective modes of therapy (Kjellberg et al. 1968, Lawrence et al. 1970a), but there were concerns regarding the incidence of damage to adjacent brain (Peck and McGovern 1966, Raskind 1967).

Radiation therapists began to recognise that pretreatment GH levels above 40–50 μg/l (80–100 mU/l) were associated with poorer outcomes (Sheline and Wara 1975). Sheline reported a reduction to <5 μg/l (<10 mU/l) by 3 years in 64% of patients with preoperative GH levels <50 μg/l (<100 mU/l), and 57% of those with preoperative levels >50 μg/l (>100 mU/l). Efficacy at 1 year was significantly lower. Radiation therapy was criticised for the long delay in producing significant reductions in GH levels. The unwanted effects of radiation therapy, such as panhypopituitarism and visual deficits, were also becoming apparent (Lamberg et al. 1976). The initial reports of less than optimal reductions in GH levels encouraged alternative treatments to be considered.

Interstitial radiation therapy

Interstitial radiation therapy was one of these modalities. Oskar Hirsch in 1921 had initially proposed interstitial radiation treatment using radium pellets held in the sphenoid sinus below an opened sella turcica. In the 1950s other investigators refined interstitial techniques using ^{198}Au and ^{90}Y to effect pituitary ablation in the treatment of diabetic retinopathy as well as breast and prostate cancer (Huggins and Bergenstal 1952, Poulsen 1953, Forrest et al. 1959, Fraser et al. 1962). In 1961 Joplin et al. reported on the first series of acromegalic patients treated with interstitial radiation. Interstitial ^{90}Y required a dose of 500 Gy, but could successfully relieve symptoms of headache and sweating, restore normal carbohydrate metabolism and improve visual fields (Wright et al. 1970, Hibbert and Shaheen 1977). Unfortunately, however, fewer than 50% of patients experienced a fall of GH to <10 μg/l (<20 mU/l) and only 30% of patients were found to have GH levels <5 μg/l (<10 mU/l; Wright et al. 1970, Hibbert and Shaheen 1977). The procedures were also complicated by cerebrospinal fluid (CSF) rhinorrhoea, cranial nerve injuries and hypopituitarism, which occurred in approximately 30% of patients (Wright et al. 1970).

Surgical history

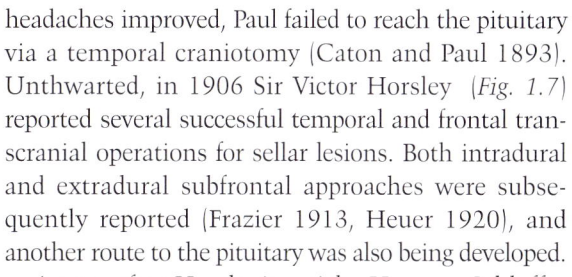

F T Paul performed the first surgical intervention for a patient with acromegaly in Liverpool in 1892 (Fig. 1.6). As reported the following year, although the patient's headaches improved, Paul failed to reach the pituitary via a temporal craniotomy (Caton and Paul 1893). Unthwarted, in 1906 Sir Victor Horsley (Fig. 1.7) reported several successful temporal and frontal transcranial operations for sellar lesions. Both intradural and extradural subfrontal approaches were subsequently reported (Frazier 1913, Heuer 1920), and another route to the pituitary was also being developed.

A year after Horsley's article, Herman Schloffer (1907) performed the first successful transsphenoidal operation for a pituitary lesion. The following year, Hochenegg (1908) reported the first successful one for acromegaly. The transsphenoidal approach sparked interest in the USA and Harvey Cushing (Fig. 1.8), for his first transsphenoidal operation, chose a 35-year-old acromegalic farmer (Figs 1.9 and 1.10) referred to him by Dr C H Mayo (Cushing 1909b).

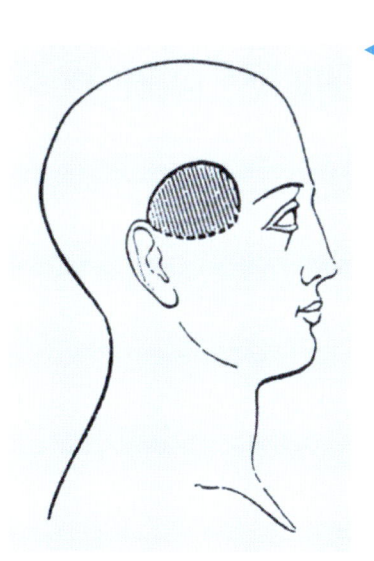

Figure 1.6 Paul's first surgical intervention for a pituitary tumour via a temporal craniotomy failed (Reproduced from *British Medical Journal*, 1893, ii, 1421–1423, with permission from the BMJ Publishing Group.)

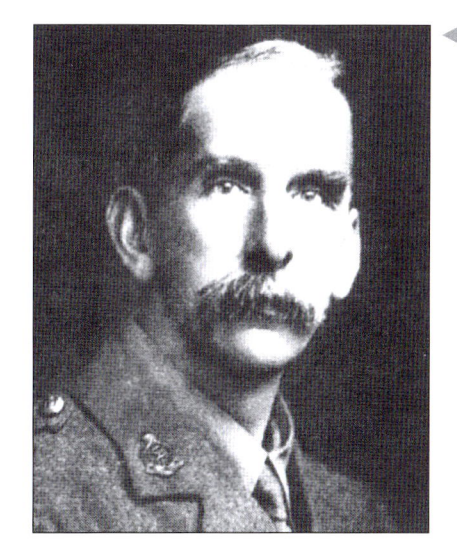

Figure 1.7 Sir Victor Horsley, 1857–1916.

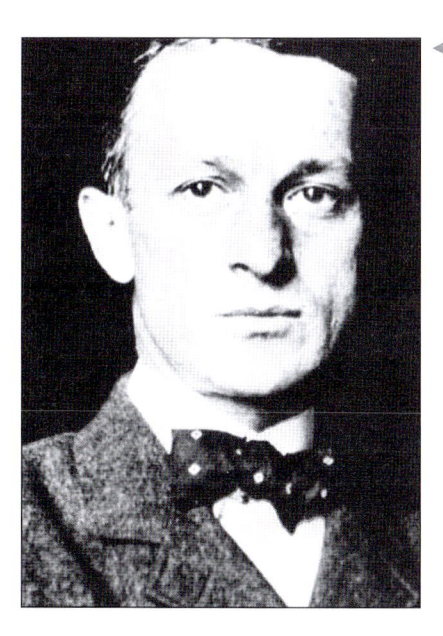

Figure 1.8 Harvey Cushing, 1869–1939.

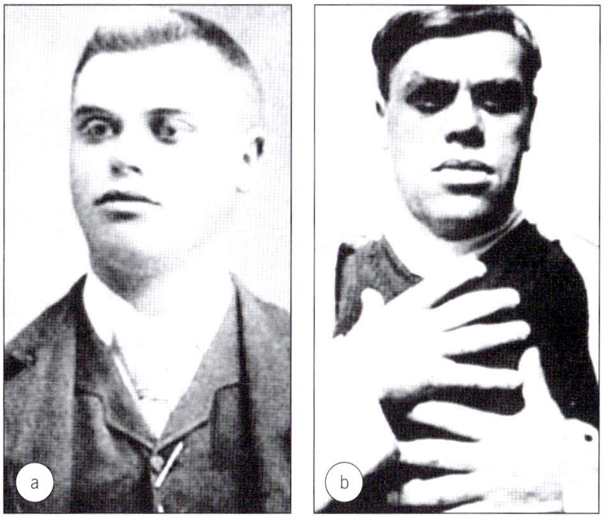

Figure 1.9 Cushing's first acromegalic patient. (a) Some years before presentation and (b) at admission.

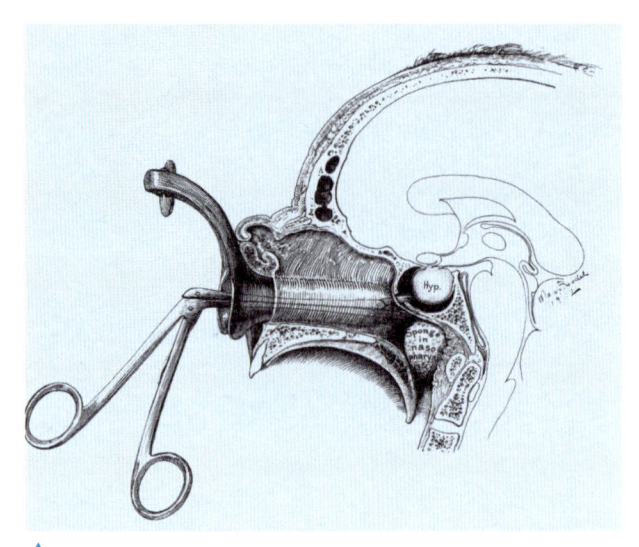

Figure 1.10 Illustration by Max Brodel of Harvey Cushing's transsphenoidal approach.

The transsphenoidal approach was initially embraced and modified (Kanavel 1909, Kocher 1909, Halstead 1910a, 1910b, Hirsch 1910). However, after over 400 transsphenoidal operations, Cushing abandoned this approach in favour of the transcranial route (Henderson 1939, Rosegay 1981). Although the precise reason for the change is not apparent, most neurosurgeons followed his lead and abandoned the transsphenoidal route. Oscar Hirsch and a pupil of Cushing, Norman Dott (*Fig. 1.11*), continued to advocate the transsphenoidal technique and taught those who would eventually revive the approach in the late 1960s.

Prior to the 1950s and 1960s, safe and successful surgery for pituitary tumours was limited by the absence of perioperative corticosteroids and antibiotics. The enlarged frontal sinus and thickened cranium of acromegalic patients made transcranial surgery for these individuals particularly challenging. Surgical intervention was restricted to patients who required rapid decompression, as when vision was threatened. Otherwise, most patients were treated with radiation and, at times, medical therapy.

However, after the introduction of corticosteroids and antibiotics, surgical approaches, regardless of the route, could be performed with significantly greater safety. By the 1960s Ray reported a low morbidity and mortality using a transfrontal approach for acromegaly (Ray and Horwith 1964, Ray *et al.* 1968). Surgeons during this time were also regaining experience with the transsphenoidal approach because of the wide application of hypophysectomy for breast carcinoma and diabetic retinopathy (Pearson *et al.* 1968). In the late 1960s and early 1970s Gerard Guiot, a pupil of Norman Dott, and Jules Hardy (*Fig. 1.12*) reintroduced the transsphenoidal approach for pituitary adenomas (Hardy and Wigser 1965, Guiot *et al.* 1967, Hardy 1967, 1969, 1971, Guiot and Derome 1972, Guiot 1973). Their use of intraoperative fluoroscopy and the operative microscope significantly facilitated transsphenoidal exposure and tumour removal. Hardy, in particular, popularised selective tumour removal while preserving the normal pituitary gland and function. Since the efficacy of radiation therapy was being questioned, the medical and neurosurgical community embraced these refinements. Early reports

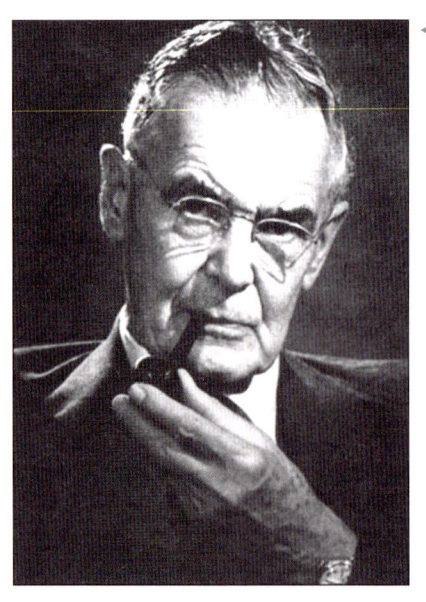

Figure 1.11 Norman Dott, 1897–1973.

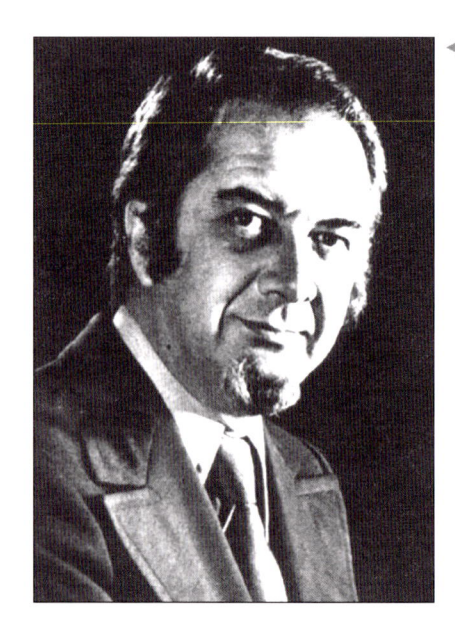

Figure 1.12 Jules Hardy.

indicated that transsphenoidal surgery could rapidly reduce GH levels to <5 µg/l (<10 mU/l) in 62–78% of patients, while producing new hormonal deficits in 26–33% (Atkinson et al. 1975, Williams et al. 1975). Results for microadenomas were quite good with 88% of patients attaining GH levels <5 µg/l (<10 mU/l) and none having new endocrine deficits (Laws et al. 1979). These early reports set the stage for the current dominant role of the transsphenoidal approach.

History of medical therapy

At the beginning of the 20th century medical therapy for acromegaly included iodine, arsenic, mercury, strychnine and caffeine. However, these treatments were unsuccessful in affecting the disease. Oestrogen therapy was alleged to produce clinical improvement and to correct aberrant carbohydrate metabolism (Kirklin and Wilder 1936, McCullagh et al. 1955). However, with the advent of the GH radioimmunoassay, oestrogen was shown not to reduce GH levels (Mintz et al. 1967, Schwartz et al. 1969).

In the late 1960s and early 1970s several groups attempted to apply the growing knowledge of the hypothalamic–pituitary axis to propose new medical treatments for acromegaly. Experiments indicated that in some patients GH secretion by an adenoma was not autonomous and, to some extent, was under hypothalamic control (Cryer and Daughaday 1969, Lawrence et al. 1970b, Nakagawa et al. 1970). Therefore drugs that disrupted the hypothalamic signals governing GH release could be used to treat acromegaly.

Medroxyprogesterone was known to act at the hypothalamic level and suppress the GH response to the insulin tolerance test (Imon et al. 1967). This medication was applied to acromegaly and, although medroxyprogesterone was shown to decrease GH levels and improve the cosmetic symptoms in some patients, the number of patients who benefited was limited (Lawrence and Kirsteins 1970, Malarkey and Doughaday 1971). Catecholamines were also shown to increase the hypothalamic stimulation of GH secretion in normal subjects (Muller et al. 1968, 1970, Boyd et al. 1970). Investigators proposed and studied whether disruption of the catecholamine effect could be used to treat acromegaly (Sherman and Kolodny 1971). Dopamine, for example, was known to increase GH secretion in Parkinson's patients (Boyd et al. 1970) and its antagonist, chlorpromazine, was tested and found to suppress GH levels in normal subjects (Sherman et al. 1971). In acromegalic patients, however, despite an apparent initial success (Kolodny et al. 1971), chlorpromazine was soon found to provide few patients either biochemical or symptomatic relief (Dimond et al. 1973). Although the alpha-adrenergic antagonist phentolamine and serotonin antagonists were shown to reduce GH levels in some acromegalic patients, only small numbers of patients improved, which limited the usefulness of these drugs (Delitala et al. 1976, Feldman et al. 1976, Nakagaws and Mashimo 1973).

In line with these clinical studies, in 1973 Hall et al. reported that parenterally administered somatostatin could reduce GH levels effectively. Although effective, somatostatin's short half-life and parenteral administration significantly limited its clinical use (Besser et al. 1974a, 1974b). In 1972, despite the knowledge that dopamine agonists raised GH levels in normal subjects, Liuzzi et al. studied its effects in acromegalic patients and reported that L-dopa paradoxically suppressed GH levels. This drug, like somatostatin, also suffered from a short half-life. Unlike somatostatin, however, a longer-acting dopamine agonist was available and Liuzzi et al. (1974a, 1974b) and coworkers were able to show significant and rapid GH suppression using bromocriptine. Soon after Luizzi's articles, Thorner reported on the first clinical series using bromocriptine and showed that the drug reduced GH levels in 80% of patients and improved both glucose tolerance and acromegalic symptoms (Thorner et al. 1975). These initial studies laid the foundation for the focus now given to medical therapy.

Other treatments

In an effort to treat patients with diabetic retinopathy and certain forms of cancer, several stereotactic ablation procedures were developed in the 1950s. Talairach and Tournoux reported the first such procedure via a transnasal approach in 1955. In 1964, Rand et al. introduced stereotactic cryohypophysectomy. These techniques were applied to acromegaly, but the results were not impressive. Whereas many patients experienced symptomatic improvement, limited numbers benefited from lower GH levels (Adams et al. 1968). The high incidence, in early reports, of rhinorrhoea occurring in 12–30% of cases (Bleasel and Lazarus 1965, Wilson et al. 1966) limited its appeal. Stereotactic radiofrequency thermal ablation was also pursued with similar results. Although modest numbers of patients experienced a fall in GH levels, early reports revealed that this procedure was also complicated by CSF leaks and meningitis (Zervas and Gordy 1967, Zervas 1969). As both cryo- and thermal hypophysectomy were designed to effect hypophyseal ablation, for acromegalic patients these procedures were associated with the undesirable attribute of a high incidence of postoperative pituitary dysfunction (Zervas and Gordy 1967).

CONCLUSION

By the mid-1970s the major hormones involved in the hypothalamic–pituitary axis (GH, somatomedins, somatostatin, GHRH) had been described. Criteria used to judge the efficacy of a given treatment modality had evolved to include a low associated morbidity, relief from mass effect and symptoms of acromegaly, maintenance of normal pituitary function and biochemical reduction in abnormal hormone levels. Although an assay for the somatomedins was still wanting, GH could be assayed and used to assess critically the outcome associated with a given treatment modality. The optimal post-treatment GH level, whether measured during fasting or after an oral glucose load, remained uncertain. Radiation therapy was known to produce moderate, albeit delayed, reductions in GH levels, but risked causing pituitary dysfunction. The transsphenoidal approach had emerged as a safe operation, one that could rapidly and effectively reduce GH levels without significant risk of new endocrine deficits. Effective medical therapy was also being pursued, and early studies had indicated a role for somatostatin analogues and dopamine agonists in the treatment of this elusive disease.

Selected readings

Elias WJ & Laws ER Jr 2000 Transsphenoidal approaches to lesions of the sella. In *Operative Neurosurgical Techniques: Indications, Methods, and Results*, 4th edn, Vol. 1, pp 373–384. Eds Schmidek HH & Sweet WH. Philadelphia: WB Saunders.

Laws ER Jr, Randall RV, Kern EB & Abboud CF (Eds) 1982 *Management of Pituitary Adenomas and Related Lesions with Emphasis on Transsphenoidal Microsurgery*. New York: Appleton–Century–Crofts.

Laws ER Jr 1996 Acromegaly and gigantism. In *Neurosurgery*, 2nd edn, Vol. 1, pp 1317–1320. Eds Wilkins RA & Rengachary SS. New York: McGraw-Hill.

Robbins RJ & Melmed S (Eds) 1987 *Acromegaly: A Century of Scientific and Clinical Progress*. New York: Plenum Press.

Wass JAH, Laws ER Jr, Randall RV & Sheline GE 1986 The treatment of acromegaly. *Clinical Endocrinology and Metabolism* **15** 683–707.

References

Adams JE, Seymour RJ, Earll JM, Tuck M, Sparks LL & Forsham PH 1968 Transsphenoidal cryohypophysectomy in acromegaly. Clinical and endocrinological evaluation. *Journal of Neurosurgery* **28** 100–104.

Anonymous 1985 Memoir on the pancreas and on the role of pancreatic juice in digestive processes, particularly in the digestion of neutral fat. By Claude Bernard. 1856. Translated by John Henderson. *Monographs of the Physiological Society* **42** 1–131.

Atkinson RL, Becker DP, Martins AN et al. 1975 Acromegaly. Treatment by transsphenoidal microsurgery. *JAMA* **233** 1279–1283.

Bayliss WM & Starling EH 1902 The mechanism of pancreatic secretion. *Journal of Physiology (London)* **28** 325–353.

Beck P, Schalch DS, Parker ML, Kipnis DM & Daughaday WH 1965 Correlative studies of growth hormone and insulin plasma concentrations with metabolic abnormalities in acromegaly. *Journal of Laboratory and Clinical Medicine* **66** 366–379.

Béclère A 1909 Le traitment médical des tumeurs hypophysaires du gigantisme et de l'acromégalie par la radio-thérapie. *Bulletins et Mémoires de la Société des Hôpitaux de Paris* **27** 274.

Benda C 1900 Beitrage zur normalen und pathologischen histologie der menschlichen hypophysis cerebri. *Klinische Wochenschrift* **52** 1205–1210.

Besser GM, Mortimer CH, Carr D et al. 1974a Growth hormone release inhibiting hormone in acromegaly. *British Medical Journal* **i** 352–355.

Besser GM, Mortimer CH, McNeilly AS et al. 1974b Long-term infusion of growth hormone release inhibiting hormone in acromegaly: effects on pituitary and pancreatic hormones. *British Medical Journal* **i** 622–627.

Bleasel K & Lazarus L 1965 Cryogenic hypophysectomy. *Medical Journal of Australia* **2** 148–150.

Boyd AE, Lebovitz HE & Pfeiffer JB 1970 Stimulation of human-growth-hormone secretion by L-dopa. *New England Journal of Medicine* **283** 1425–1429.

Brazeau P, Vale W, Burgus R et al. 1973 Hypothalamic polypeptide that inhibits the secretion of immunoreactive pituitary growth hormone. *Science* **179** 77–79.

Brigidi V 1881 Studii anatomo-patologici sopra un uomo divenuto stranamente deforme per cronica infermita. *Archivo di Scuola Anatomie e Patologia di Universita di Firenze* 65–92.

Brissaud E & Meige H 1895 Gigantisme et acromégalie. *Revue Scientifique* **3** 575.

Caton R, Paul, FT 1893 Notes on a case of acromegaly treated by operation. *British Medical Journal* **ii** 1421–1423.

Cryer PE, Daughaday WH 1969 Regulation of growth hormone secretion in acromegaly. *Journal of Clinical Endocrinology and Metabolism* **29** 386–393.

Cushing H 1909a The hypophysis cerebri: clinical aspects of hyperpituitarism and of hypopituitarism. *JAMA* **53** 249–255.

Cushing H 1909b Partial hypophysectomy for acromegaly. *Annals of Surgery* **50** 1002–1017.

Cushing H 1909c Partial hypophysectomy for acromegaly: with remarks on the function of the hypophysis. *Annals of Surgery* **50** 1002–1017.

Cushing H 1912 *The Pituitary Body and its Disorders*. Philadelphia: JB Lippincott Co.

Daughaday WH, Salmon WD Jr & Alexander F 1959 Sulfation factor activity of sera from patients with pituitary disorders. *Journal of Clinical Endocrinology and Metabolism* **19** 743–758.

Daughaday WH, Hall K, Raben MS, Salmon WD Jr, van den Brande JL & van Wyk JJ 1972 Somatomedin: proposed designation for sulphation factor. *Nature* **235** 107.

Delitala G, Masala A, Alagna S, Devilla L & Lotti G 1976 Growth hormone and prolactin release in acromegalic patients following metergoline administration. *Journal of Clinical Endocrinology and Metabolism* **43** 1382–1386.

Deuben RR & Meites J 1964 Simulation of pituitary growth hormone release by a hypothalamic extract *in vitro*. *Endocrinology* **74** 408–409.

Dimond RC, Bramer SR, Atkinson RL, Howard WJ & Earll JM 1973 Chlorpromazine treatment and growth hormone secretory responses in acromegaly. *Journal of Clinical Endocrinology and Metabolism* **36** 1189–1195.

Du Bois Reymond E 1877 *Gesammelte Abhandlungen zur allgemeinen Muskel und Nerven Physic*, Vol. 2. Leipzig: Veit & Co.

Ellis S, Huble J & Simpson ME 1953 Influence of hypophysectomy and growth hormone on cartilage sulfate metabolism. *Proceedings of the Society for Experimental Biology and Medicine* **84** 603–605.

Evans HM & Long JA 1921 The effect of the anterior lobe of the pituitary administered intra-peritoneally upon growth, maturity and oestrus cycle of the rat. *The Anatomical Record* **21** 62.

Feldman JM, Plonk JW & Bivens CH 1976 Inhibitory effect of serotonin antagonists on growth hormone release in acromegalic patients. *Clinical Endocrinology (Oxford)* **5** 71–78.

Forrest APM & Peebles-Brown DA. 1955 Pituitary radon implant for breast. *Lancet* **i** 1054–1055.

Fraser R, Joplin GF & Steiner RE 1962 Pituitary ablation by yttrium-90 implants for diabetic retinopathy. *Diabetes* **11** 482–483.

Frazier CH 1913 An approach to the hypophysis through the anterior cranial fossa. *Annals of Surgery* **57** 145–150.

Freud J, Levine LH & Kroon DB 1939 Observations on growth (chondrotrophic) hormone and localization of its point of attack. *Journal of Endocrinology* **1** 56–64.

Furlanetto RW, Underwood L, Van Wyk JJ & D'Ercole AJ 1977 Estimation of somatomedin-C levels in normals and patients with pituitary disease by radioimmunoassay. *Journal of Clinical Investigation* **60** 648–657.

Glick SM, Roth J, Yalow RS & Berson SA 1963 Immunoassay of human growth hormone in plasma. *Nature* **199** 784–787.

Gramegna A 1909 Un cas d'acromégalie traité par la radiothérapie. *Revue Neurologie* **17** 15–17.

Guillemin R, Brazeau P, Bohlen P, Esch F, Ling N & Wehrenberg WB 1982 Growth hormone-releasing factor from a human pancreatic tumor that caused acromegaly. *Science* **218** 585–587.

Guiot G 1973 Transsphenoidal approach in surgical treatment of pituitary adenomas: general principles and indications in nonfunctioning adenomas. In *Diagnosis and Treatment of Pituitary Tumors*, pp 159–178. Eds Kohler PO & Ross GT. New York: American Elsevier.

Guiot G & Derome P 1972 [Indications for trans-sphenoidal approach in neurosurgery. 521 cases]. *Annales de Médecine Interne (Paris)* **123** 703–712.

Guiot G, Bouche J & Oproiu A 1967 [Indications of the trans-sphenoidal approach to pituitary adenomas. Experience with 165 operations]. *Presse Médicale* **75** 1563–1568.

Hall R, Besser GM, Schally AV et al. 1973 Action of growth-hormone-release inhibitory hormone in healthy men and in acromegaly. *Lancet* **ii** 581–584.

Halstead AE 1910a The operative treatment of tumors of the hypophysis. *Surgery, Gynecology and Obstetrics* **10** 494.

Halstead AE 1910b Remarks on the operative treatment of tumors of the hypophysis. With the report of two cases operated on by an oronasal method. *Transactions of the American Surgical Association* **28** 73–93.

Hardy J 1967 [Surgery of the pituitary gland, using the trans-sphenoidal approach. Comparative study of 2 technical methods]. *Union Médicale du Canada* **96** 702–712.

Hardy J 1969 Transsphenoidal microsurgery of the normal and pathological pituitary. *Clinical Neurosurgery* **16** 185–217.

Hardy J 1971 Transsphenoidal hypophysectomy. *Journal of Neurosurgery* **34** 582–594.

Hardy J & Wigser SM 1965 Trans-sphenoidal surgery of pituitary fossa tumors with televised radiofluoroscopic control. *Journal of Neurosurgery* **23** 612–619.

Henderson WR 1939 The pituitary adenomata. A follow-up study of the surgical results in 338 cases (Dr Harvey Cushing's series). *British Journal of Surgery* **26** 911–921.

Heuer GJ 1920 Surgical experiences with an intracranial approach to chiasmal lesions. *Archives of Surgery* **1** 369–381.

Hibbert J & Shaheen OH 1977 The treatment of acromegaly by yttrium implantation. *Journal of Laryngology and Otology* **91** 1–9.

Hirsch O 1910 Endonasal method of removal of hypophyseal tumors. *JAMA* **5** 772–774.

Hirsch O 1921 Radiumbehandlung der Hypophysentumoren. *Archiv für Laryngologie und Rhinologie* **34** 133–148.

Hochenegg J 1908 Operat geheilte Akromegalie bei Hypophysentumor. *Langenbecks Archiv für Chirurgie. Supplement II. Verhandlungen der Deutschen Gesellschaft für Chirurgie* **37** 80–85.

Horsley V 1906 Address in surgery on the technic of operation on the central nervous system. *British Medical Journal* **ii** 411–423.

Huggins C & Bergenstal DM 1952 Inhibition of human mammary and prostatic cancers by adrenalectomy. *Cancer Research* **12** 131–141.

Hunter WM & Greenwood FC 1962 Preparation of iodine-131 labelled human growth hormone in plasma. *Nature* **194** 495–496.

Imon S, Schiffer M, Glick SM & Schwartz E 1967 Effect of medroxyprogesterone acetate upon stimulated release of growth hormone in men. *Journal of Clinical Endocrinology and Metabolism* **27** 1633–1636.

Jae Lee P 1970 *Giant: The Pictorial History of the Human Colossus*. Cranbury: AS Barnes & Co.

Joplin GF, Frazer R, Steiner R, Laws J & Jones E 1961 Partial pituitary ablation by needle implantation of gold-198 seeds for acromegaly and Cushing's disease. *Lancet* **ii** 1277–1280.

Kanavel AB 1909 The removal of tumors of the pituitary body by an infranasal route. *JAMA* **53** 1704–1707.

Kinsell LW, Michaels GD, Li CH & Larsen W 1947 Studies in growth. I. Interrelationship between pituitary growth factor and growth promoting androgens in acromegaly and gigantism. II. Quantitative evaluation of bone and soft tissue growth in acromegaly and gigantism. *Journal of Clinical Endocrinology and Metabolism* **8** 1013–1036.

Kirklin OL & Wilder RM 1936 Follicular hormone administered in acromegaly. *Mayo Clinic Proceedings* **11** 121–125.

Kjellberg RN, Shintani A, Frantz AG & Kliman B 1968 Proton-beam therapy in acromegaly. *New England Journal of Medicine* **278** 689–695.

Kocher T 1909 Ein Fall von Hypophysis-Tumor mit operativer Heilung. *Deutscher Zeitschrift für Mund-, Kiefer- und Gesichts-Chirurgie* **100** 13–37.

Kolodny HD, Sherman L, Singh A, Kim S & Benjamin F 1971 Acromegaly treated with chlorpromazine. A case study. *New England Journal of Medicine* **284** 819–822.

Kramer S 1973 Indications for, and results of, treatment of pituitary tumors by external radiation. In *Diagnosis and Treatment of Pituitary Tumors*, pp 217–233. Eds Kohler PO & Ross GT. New York: American Elsevier.

Krulich L, Dhariwal AP & McCann S 1968 Stimulatory and inhibitory effects of purified hypothalamic extracts on growth hormone release from rat pituitary *in vitro*. *Endocrinology* **83** 783–790.

Lamberg BA, Kivikangas V, Vartianen J, Raitta C & Pelkonen R 1976 Conventional pituitary irradiation in acromegaly. Effect on growth hormone and TSH secretion. *Acta Endocrinologica (Copenhagen)* **82** 267–281.

Lawrence AM and Kirsteins L 1970 Progestins in the medical management of active acromegaly. *Journal of Clinical Endocrinology and Metabolism* **30** 646–652.

Lawrence JH, Tobias CA, Born JL, Sangalli R, Carlson RA & Linfoot JH 1962 Heavy particle therapy in acromegaly. *Acta Radiologica* **58** 337–347.

Lawrence JH, Tobias CA, Linfoot JA et al. 1970a Successful treatment of acromegaly: metabolic and clinical studies in 145 patients. *Journal of Clinical Endocrinology and Metabolism* **31** 180–198.

Lawrence AM, Goldfine ID & Kirsteins L 1970b Growth hormone dynamics in acromegaly. *Journal of Clinical Endocrinology and Metabolism* **31** 239–247.

Lawrence AM, Pinsky SM & Goldfine ID 1971 Conventional radiation therapy in acromegaly. A review and reassessment. *Archives of Internal Medicine* **128** 369–377.

Laws ER Jr, Piepgras DG, Randall RV & Abboud CF 1979 Neurosurgical management of acromegaly. Results in 82 patients treated between 1972 and 1977. *Journal of Neurosurgery* **50** 454–461.

Ling N, Burgus R, Rivier J, Vale W & Brazeau P 1973 The use of mass spectrometry in deducing the sequence of somatostatin – a hypothalamic polypeptide that inhibits the secretion of growth hormone. *Biochemical and Biophysical Research Communications* **50** 127–133.

Liuzzi A, Chiodini PG, Botalla L, Cremascoli G & Silvestrini F 1972 Inhibitory effect of L-dopa on GH release in acromegalic patients. *Journal of Clinical Endocrinology and Metabolism* **35** 941–943.

Liuzzi A, Chiodini PG, Botalla L, Cremascoli G, Muller EE & Silvestrini F 1974a Decreased plasma growth hormone (GH) levels in acromegalics following CB 154 (2-Br-alpha ergocryptine) administration. *Journal of Clinical Endocrinology and Metabolism* **38** 910–912.

Liuzzi A, Chiodini PG, Botalla L, Silvestrini F & Muller EE 1974b Growth hormone (GH)-releasing activity of TRH and GH-lowering effect of dopaminergic drugs in acromegaly: homogeneity in the two responses. *Journal of Clinical Endocrinology and Metabolism* **39** 871–876.

Malarkey WB & Daughaday WH 1971 Variable response of plasma GH in acromegalic patients treated with medroxyprogesterone acetate. *Journal of Clinical Endocrinology and Metabolism* **33** 424–431.

Marie P 1886 Sur deux cas d'acromégalie: hypertrophie singulière, non congénitale, des extrémités supérieures, inférieures et céphalique. *Revue Médicale de Liege* **6** 297–333.

Marie P & Marinesco G 1891 Sur l'anatomie pathologique de l'acromégalie. *Archives de Médecine Expérimentale et d'Anatomie Pathologique* **3** 539–565.

Massalongo R 1892 Sull'acromegalia. *Riforma Medica* **8** 74–77.

McCullagh EP, Beck JC & Schaffenburg CA 1955 Control of diabetes and other features of acromegaly following treatment with estrogens. *Diabetes* **4** 13–23.

Mintz DH, Finster JL & Josimovich JB 1967 Effect of estrogen therapy on carbohydrate metabolism in acromegaly. *Journal of Clinical Endocrinology and Metabolism* **27** 1321–1327.

Muller EE, Dal Pra P & Pecile A 1968 Influence of brain neurohumors injected into the lateral ventricle of the rat on growth hormone release. *Endocrinology* **83** 893–896.

Muller EE, Pecile A, Felici M & Cocchi D 1970 Norepinephrine and dopamine injection into lateral brain ventricle of the rat and growth hormone-releasing activity in the hypothalamus and plasma. *Endocrinology* **86** 1376–1382.

Murphy WR, Daughaday WH & Hartnett C 1956 The effect of hypophysectomy and growth hormone on the incorporation of labeled sulfate into tibial epiphyseal and nasal cartilage of the rat. *Journal of Laboratory and Clinical Medicine* **47** 715–221.

Nakagawa K & Mashimo K 1973 Suppressibility of plasma growth hormone levels in acromegaly with dexamethasone and phentolamine. *Journal of Clinical Endocrinology and Metabolism* **37** 238–246.

Nakagawa K, Horiuchi Y & Mashimo K 1970 Effect of dexamethasone on plasma growth hormone levels in acromegaly. *Journal of Clinical Endocrinology and Metabolism* **31** 502–506.

Niall HD, Hogan ML, Tregear GW, Segre GV, Hwang P & Friesen H 1973 The chemistry of growth hormone and the lactogenic hormones. *Recent Progress in Hormone Research* **29** 387–416.

Pearson OH, Thomas CH, Kaufman B et al. 1968 Pituitary ablation in the treatment of diabetic retinopathy. In *Symposium on Treatment of Diabetic Retinopathy*, Public Health Service Publication No. 1890, pp 331–339. Eds Goldberg MF & Find SL Warrenton, Virginia: Government Printing Office.

Peck FC Jr & McGovern ER 1966 Radiation necrosis of the brain in acromegaly. *Journal of Neurosurgery* **25** 536–542.

Pistenma DA, Goffinet DR, Bagshaw MA, Hanbery JW & Eltringham JR 1976 Treatment of acromegaly with megavoltage radiation therapy. *International Journal of Radiation Oncology, Biology, Physics* **1** 885–893.

Poulsen JE 1953 Houssay phenomenon in man: recovery from retinopathy in case of diabetes with Simmonds' disease. *Diabetes* **2** 7–12.

Quabbe HJ, Schilling E & Helge H 1966 Pattern of growth hormone secretion during a 24-hour fast in normal adults. *Journal of Clinical Endocrinology and Metabolism* **26** 1173–1177.

Raben MS 1957 Preparation of growth hormone from pituitaries of man and monkey. *Science* **125** 883–884.

Rand RW, Dashe AM, Paglia DE, Conway LW & Solomon DH 1964 Stereotactic cryohypophysectomy. *JAMA* **189** 255–259.

Raskind R 1967 Central nervous system damage after radiation therapy. *International Surgery* **48** 430–441.

Ray BS & Horwith M 1964 Surgical treatment of acromegaly. *Clinical Neurosurgery* **10** 31–59.

Ray BS, Horwith M & Mautalen C 1968 Surgical hypophysectomy as a treatment for acromegaly. In *Clinical Endocrinology*, pp 93–102. Eds Astwood EB & Cassidy CE. New York: Grune & Stratton.

Reichlin S 1960 Growth and the hypothalamus. *Endocrinology* **67** 760–773.

Rivier J, Spiess J, Thorner M & Vale W 1982 Characterization of a growth hormone-releasing factor from a human pancreatic islet tumour. *Nature* **300** 276–278.

Rosegay H 1981 Cushing's legacy to transsphenoidal surgery. *Journal of Neurosurgery* **54** 448–454.

Roth J, Glick SM, Yalow RS & Berson SA 1963 Stimulation of pituitary growth hormone release by a hypothalamic extract *in vitro*. *Science* **140** 987–988.

Roth J, Glick SM & Hollander CS 1967 Acromegaly and other disorders of growth hormone secretion. *Annals of Internal Medicine* **66** 760–788.

Roth J, Gorden P & Brace K 1970 Efficacy of conventional pituitary irradiation in acromegaly. *New England Journal of Medicine* **282** 1385–1391.

Salmon WD Jr & Daughaday WH 1957 A hormonally controlled serum factor which stimulates sulfate incorporation by cartilage *in vitro*. *Journal of Laboratory and Clinical Medicine* **49** 825–836.

Schloffer H 1907 Erfolgreiche Operationen eines Hypophentamors auf Nasalem Wage. *Wiener Klinische Wochenschrift* **20** 621–624.

Schwartz E, Echemendia E, Schiffer M & Panariello VA 1969 Mechanism of estrogenic action in acromegaly. *Journal of Clinical Investigation* **48** 260–270.

Sheline GE, Goldberg MB & Feldman R 1961 Pituitary irradiation for acromegaly. *Radiology* **76** 70–75.

Sheline GE & Wara WM 1975 Radiation therapy for acromegaly and nonsecretory chromophobe adenomas of the pituitary. In *Tumors of the Nervous System*, pp 117–132. Ed Seydel HG. New York: John Wiley.

Sherman L & Kolodny HD 1971 The hypothalamus, brain-catecholamines, and drug therapy for gigantism and acromegaly. *Lancet* **i** 682–685.

Sherman L, Kim S, Benjamin F & Kolodny HD 1971 Effect of chlorpromazine on serum growth-hormone concentration in man. *New England Journal of Medicine* **284** 72–74.

Smith PE 1927 The disabilities caused by hypophysectomy and their repair. *JAMA* **83** 158–161.

Takahashi Y, Kipnis DM & Daughaday WH 1968 Growth hormone secretion during sleep. *Journal of Clinical Investigation* **47** 2079–2090.

Talairach J & Tournoux P 1955 Appareil de stéréotaxie hypophysaire pour voie d'abord nasale. *Neuro-chirurgie* **1** 127–131.

Thorner MO, Chait A, Aitken M *et al*. 1975 Bromocriptine treatment of acromegaly. *British Medical Journal* **i** 299–303.

Utiger RD, Parker ML & Daughaday WH 1962 Studies on human growth hormone: a radioimmunoassay for human growth hormone. *Journal of Clinical Investigation* **41** 254–261.

Verga A 1864 Caso singolare di prosopectasia. *Rendiconti (Reale Istituto 1st Lombardo di Scienze e Lettere. Classe di Scienze Matematiche e Naturali)* **1** 111–117.

von Mering JV & Minkowski O 1889 Diabetes Mellitus nach Pankreasexstirpation. *Zentralblatt für Klinische Medizin* **10** 393.

Williams RA, Jacobs HS, Kurtz AB *et al*. 1975 The treatment of acromegaly with special reference to trans-sphenoidal hypophysectomy. *Quarterly Journal of Medicine* **44** 79–98.

Wilson CB, Winternitz WW, Bertan V & Sizemore G 1966 Stereotaxic cryosurgery of the pituitary gland in carcinoma of the breast and other disorders. *JAMA* **198** 587–590.

Wright AD, Hartog M, Palter H *et al*. 1970 The use of yttrium-90 implantation in the treatment of acromegaly. *Proceedings of the Royal Society of Medicine* **63** 221–223.

Zervas NT 1969 Stereotaxic radiofrequency surgery of the normal and the abnormal pituitary gland. *New England Journal of Medicine* **280** 429–437.

Zervas NT & Gordy PD 1967 Radiofrequency hypophysectomy for metastatic breast and prostatic carcinoma. *Surgical Clinics of North America* **47** 1279–1285.

2

CLINICAL FEATURES, INVESTIGATION AND COMPLICATIONS OF ACROMEGALY

2 CLINICAL FEATURES, INVESTIGATION AND COMPLICATIONS OF ACROMEGALY

Helen E Turner Department of Endocrinology, Radcliffe Infirmary, Oxford, UK

■ EPIDEMIOLOGY

Acromegaly is a rare condition with a prevalence of about 60 cases per million population and an incidence of 3.3 new cases per year. The incidence in males and females is equal and it has been described in most racial groups. The mean age of diagnosis is between 40 and 50 years, although excessive growth hormone (GH) secretion leading to gigantism in children and acromegaly in adults occurs at all ages. The average delay in diagnosis from onset of symptoms is estimated to be approximately 8 years.

■ MORTALITY

Acromegaly leads to a reduced life expectancy, with an increase in mortality rate between two- and four-fold. From several retrospective cohort studies, the predominant determinant of outcome is the most recent serum GH concentration (Rajasoorya et al. 1994, Orme et al. 1998, Swearingen et al. 1998). Elevated insulin-like growth factor-I (IGF-I) is also associated with increased mortality (Swearingen et al. 1998).

Other factors associated with increased mortality include duration of symptoms prior to diagnosis, duration of disease, older age at diagnosis and the presence of cardiovascular disease, diabetes and hypertension at diagnosis (Wright et al. 1970, Bates et al. 1993, Rajasoorya et al. 1994, Orme et al. 1998).

Importantly, these studies also demonstrate that a reduction in GH levels is associated with reduced mortality. Patients with post-treatment GH concentrations <5 mU/l (<2.5 μg/l; Box 2.1) have a similar mortality rate to that of the general population (Bates et al. 1993, Orme et al. 1998).

Box 2.1 Note on units for growth hormone

Concentrations of GH may be measured in mU/l or μg/l. The equivalent ratio of mU/l to μg/l was previously considered to be two (as in this book) and now three (see p. xiii).

The major causes of death are cardiovascular and respiratory disease or malignancy (Table 2.1). The increased risk of malignancy has been debated, but the majority of studies demonstrate an increased risk of colon and possibly breast cancer in particular. The effect of GH deficiency on long-term mortality in patients with 'cured' acromegaly requires investigation, and it is currently unknown whether GH replacement therapy is beneficial in this group.

■ PATHOGENESIS

The clinical syndrome and complications of acromegaly result from prolonged hypersecretion of GH and of excessive IGF-I production. The most

Table 2.1 Causes of death in patients with acromegaly.

CAUSES OF DEATH IN PATIENTS WITH ACROMEGALY					
Reference	Number of deaths	Cardiovascular (%)	Cerebrovascular (%)	Respiratory (%)	Cancer (%)
Wright et al. 1970	54	24	15	19	19
Nabarro 1987	47	40	15	6	23
Bates et al. 1993	28	57 (vascular)		25	9
Rajasoorya et al. 1994	32	37	12	12	23
Orme et al. 1998	366	37	12	12	23
Swearingen et al. 1998	12	42		8	33

CAUSES OF ACROMEGALY

Condition (frequency)	Types
Pituitary adenoma (98%)	Somatotroph adenoma (sparsely granulated, densely granulated) Mammosomatotroph adenoma Acidophil stem-cell adenomas Plurihormonal adenomas (GH, prolactin and thyroid-stimulating hormone)
Pituitary carcinoma	
Ectopic GH-releasing hormone	Intracranial, e.g. hypothalamic hamartoma and gangliocytoma Extracranial, e.g. carcinoid tumour (pancreas, bronchus, gastrointestinal tract)
Ectopic GH	Intracranial, e.g. somatotrophinoma arising from embryological remnant Extracranial, e.g. pancreatic, breast or lung tumour

Table 2.2 Causes of acromegaly.

common cause of acromegaly is a benign GH-secreting pituitary adenoma (Table 2.2). Approximately one-third of patients with acromegaly are also hyperprolactinaemic because of prolactin (PRL) co-secretion from a tumour or as a result of the loss of dopamine inhibition of PRL secretion through pituitary stalk compression. Very rarely acromegaly results from a pituitary carcinoma or somatotroph hyperplasia caused by an excess of GH-releasing hormone (GHRH) secretion from both intracranial sources (such as hypothalamic hamartomas) and extracranial tumours (including carcinoid tumours of the lung, pancreas and upper gastrointestinal tract). Ectopic GH hypersecretion is very rare, and may result from intracranial sources (such as a somatotrophinoma that arises from an embryonic remnant) or from a pancreatic islet or bronchial tumour.

Several rare heritable syndromes are associated with acromegaly (Table 2.3).

The molecular basis of pituitary adenoma formation is largely unknown. It is likely that the development of pituitary adenomas is a multistep process in which genetic changes lead to dysregulated monoclonal expansion of a mutated cell. Hypothalamic hormones and local growth factors probably play a role in promoting further growth. Final tumour phenotype probably results from the interaction of various genetic changes (both activating and inactivating) with the local hypothalamic endocrine factors and paracrine growth factors.

HEREDITARY SYNDROMES ASSOCIATED WITH ACROMEGALY

Syndrome	Genetic defect	Features
McCune–Albright	Activating mutation of Gs alpha gene	Polyostotic fibrous dysplasia Hyperpigmented patches Precocious puberty Gigantism or acromegaly Cushing's syndrome
Multiple endocrine neoplasia (MEN) type 1	Autosomal dominant Inactivation of MEN 1 gene on 11q13	Primary hyperparathyroidism Pituitary adenomas Pancreatic endocrine tumours
Familial acromegaly	Autosomal dominant Loss of heterozygosity (LOH) on 11q13 (distinct from MEN 1 locus LOH on 2p16)	At least two cases of acromegaly in a family that does not exhibit MEN 1 or Carney complex
Carney syndrome	Autosomal dominant Gene(s) mapped to 2p16 by linkage analysis	Spotty mucocutaneous pigmentation Skin, cardiac and breast myxomas Pituitary adenomas (GH most commonly) Primary pigmented nodular adrenocortical disease (adrenocorticotrophin-independent Cushing's syndrome)

Table 2.3 Hereditary syndromes associated with acromegaly.

Oncogenes associated with GH-secreting pituitary adenomas (activating genetic mutations)

Activating genetic mutations lead to gain of function and are dominant at the cellular level. Therefore only one copy of the mutation is required.

Mutation of the stimulatory G protein

Mutation of the stimulatory G protein (gsp) occurs in up to 40% of human GH-secreting pituitary adenomas. Although it is the most common mutation thus far associated with somatotroph adenomas, it is rarely demonstrated in other tumour types, including non-functioning adenomas (<10%) and adrenocorticotrophin (ACTH)-secreting tumours (<6%). There is an ethnic difference in prevalence, with lower frequencies in Japanese patients (<10%).

Mutations of gsp lead to inhibition of the intrinsic guanosine triphosphatase activity on the alpha-subunit of the adenyl cyclase stimulatory G protein Gs. This results in persistent Gs activation of adenyl cyclase, which mimics persistent GHRH receptor activation and leads to autonomous GH secretion and somatotroph hyperplasia. Although there are no differences in tumour phenotype between gsp-positive and gsp-negative tumours, the former are more sensitive to treatment with somatostatin analogues.

Activated cAMP–response element binding proteins

Increased levels of activated cAMP–response element binding protein (CREB) have been demonstrated within GH-secreting pituitary adenomas, and may activate the adenyl cyclase pathway that leads to GH hypersecretion and somatotroph proliferation (Bertherat *et al.* 1995).

Pituitary tumour transforming gene

The recently described pituitary tumour transforming gene (PTTG) may play a role in pituitary tumour transformation and development. Increased PTTG mRNA occurs in pituitary adenomas compared with control pituitary glands, and expression of PTTG is positively correlated with tumour grade (Zhang *et al.* 1999).

Tumour suppressor genes associated with GH-secreting pituitary adenomas (inactivating genetic alterations)

Loss of heterozygosity (LOH) has been used to identify the chromosomal location of candidate genes. In several regions, although LOH has been demonstrated the gene defect remains unelucidated, as for 13q14, 11q13 (multiple endocrine neoplasia 1 (MEN 1) gene ruled out), 9p and 1p35.

Retinoblastoma gene

Mice with retinoblastoma gene (Rb) mutations develop pro-opiomelanocortin (POMC) tumours, but although LOH has been demonstrated at the Rb locus in humans, the presence of intact Rb protein suggests that this is a marker for a different as yet unidentified tumour suppressor gene.

Protein 53

Protein 53 (p53) mutations are not detected in the majority of pituitary adenomas, but p53 expression appears to be related to tumour aggressiveness. However, allelic loss of the functionally and structurally similar p73 (located on 1p36) was demonstrated recently.

Cyclin-dependent kinase inhibitors

Cyclin-dependent kinase (CDK) inhibitors are proteins that regulate the cell cycle, and alterations in the function of CDK inhibitors (such as p16 and p27) have been reported in some studies.

Hypothalamic factors

The role of GHRH may be autocrine or paracrine in GH-secreting adenoma pathogenesis. Overexpression of the GHRH gene has been associated with increased risk of neoplastic progression and tumour aggressiveness. In animal models of GHRH overexpression in mice, tumour formation may result. However, in humans ectopic GHRH overstimulation does not appear to lead to adenoma formation. Although as yet no evidence indicates activating mutations of GHRH receptors, some adenomas express a truncated GHRH receptor of uncertain pathophysiological significance.

In contrast to the stimulatory effect of GHRH, somatostatin exerts an inhibitory influence on GH secretion. Differences in somatostatin expression might be expected to influence GH secretion, and the lack of somatostatin in GH-secreting adenomas may therefore be important. Alterations in the expression of somatostatin-receptor subtypes in different GH-secreting adenomas change the response to somatostatin analogues, but they are not associated with differences in tumour behaviour.

The role of growth factors, such as transforming growth factor-alpha, epidermal growth factor, basic fibroblast growth factor and vascular endothelial growth factor, is currently not known. However, it is likely that some or all of these factors may play a role in the development of the GH-secreting adenoma.

HISTOPATHOLOGY

Pituitary adenomas

Pituitary adenomas can be classified (Asa and Kovacs 1992) according to size (microadenomas <10 mm in diameter or macroadenomas >10 mm in diameter), immunostain (GH, GH/PRL, plurihormonal), ultrastructure (sparsely granulated, densely granulated, mammosomatotroph tumours, acidophil stem cell) or behaviour (invasive, recurrent or metastatic).

Somatotroph adenomas are almost always associated with clinical evidence of excess GH secretion. However, rarely these tumours may be 'silent' in that GH-positive immunostaining is not associated with acromegaly or gigantism because of either an altered bioactivity of GH or the lack of detectable GH release.

Plurihormonal tumours in patients with acromegaly are most commonly GH and PRL tumours. In some patients these are mixed somatotroph–lactotroph adenomas in which discrete populations of GH and PRL secretory cells occur. In contrast, the mammosomatotroph tumours are composed of a monomorphous collection of tumour cells that produce both GH and PRL. The acidophil stem-cell adenoma is also a monomorphous GH and PRL co-secreting tumour, although PRL secretion predominates. Mixed somatotroph and thyrotroph tumours, or tumours composed of cells that co-secrete GH and thyroid-stimulating hormone (TSH), are associated with acromegaly and thyrotoxicosis. Positive immunostaining for the alpha subunit may also be found in GH-secreting tumours.

The GH-secreting tumours may be invasive, which results in bony erosion and invasion into the adjacent cavernous sinus. Tumours removed from younger patients are characteristically more likely to be macroadenomas, associated with higher GH concentrations and more aggressive tumour behaviour. Pituitary carcinomas are very rare and are diagnosed only when there is evidence of distant metastasis. This may be distant intracranial sites or extracranial sites (including lymph nodes, liver and lung). On histopathological examination of the primary tumour no abnormalities allow diagnosis of carcinoma, although nuclear pleomorphism and increased mitoses raise the suspicion of an aggressive phenotype.

Somatotroph hyperplasia develops secondary to GHRH hypersecretion. It is characterised by the lack of a distinct adenoma, enlarged acini and maintenance of the reticulin pattern.

CLINICAL FEATURES

The clinical features of acromegaly include those of GH and IGF-I on tissues and the effects of the pituitary tumour itself (Table 2.4). Local effects particularly occur in younger patients with aggressive,

CLINICAL FEATURES OF ACROMEGALY
Direct effects of tumour
Headache
Visual impairment
Hyperprolactinaemia
Hypopituitarism
Pituitary apoplexy (rare)
Soft tissue and skin changes
Acral enlargement and soft-tissue enlargement
Increased sweating
Skin tags and acanthosis nigricans
Cardiac features
Increased left ventricular mass and left ventricular hypertrophy
Biventricular failure
Ischaemic heart disease
Hypertension
Carbohydrate intolerance
Insulin resistance
Impaired glucose tolerance
Diabetes mellitus
Respiratory disease
Upper airway obstruction
Macroglossia
Obstructive sleep apnoea
Thickening of vocal chords and enlargement of tissues
Neoplasia
Colonic polyps and carcinoma
Breast, thyroid or prostate cancer?
Bone, joint and neuromuscular disorders
Joint stiffness
Arthropathy, leading to osteoarthritis
Carpal tunnel syndrome
Proximal myopathy
Osteopenia
Other endocrine dysfunction
Multinodular goitre
Hypercalciuria
Hyperparathyroidism

▲ Table 2.4 Clinical features of acromegaly.

CLINICAL FEATURES, INVESTIGATION AND COMPLICATIONS OF ACROMEGALY

rapidly growing tumours. The gradual nature of the development of the clinical features makes it important to examine any available photographs to determine the duration of disease.

Direct effects of tumour mass

The direct effects of tumour mass include headache, which may be present in up to 50% of cases at diagnosis. Visual impairment may result from the loss of visual fields, which leads to uni- or bitemporal hemianopia, and/or from a reduction in visual acuity through optic atrophy. Pituitary apoplexy (haemorrhagic infarction of the pituitary tumour) is a rare presentation of acromegaly.

Hyperprolactinaemia occurs in approximately one-third of patients and gonadotrophin deficiency is also relatively common. These factors lead to menstrual disturbance and galactorrhoea, erectile impotence and infertility. Deficiencies of ACTH and TSH are less common at presentation (<20%).

Soft-tissue and skin changes

The majority of patients at presentation have evidence of acral enlargement and soft-tissue enlargement caused by the deposition of mucopolysaccharides (Molitch 1992). Collagen production is also increased. Typical features include enlarged doughy hands and feet, coarsening of facial features with prognathism, jaw malocclusion, frontal bossing, thickened lips and facial skin folds (*Figs 2.1–2.3*). These exaggerated skin folds may be visible on a skull radiograph and are known as 'cutis verticis gyrata'. Increased sweating is very common. These changes are reversible with treatment to lower the

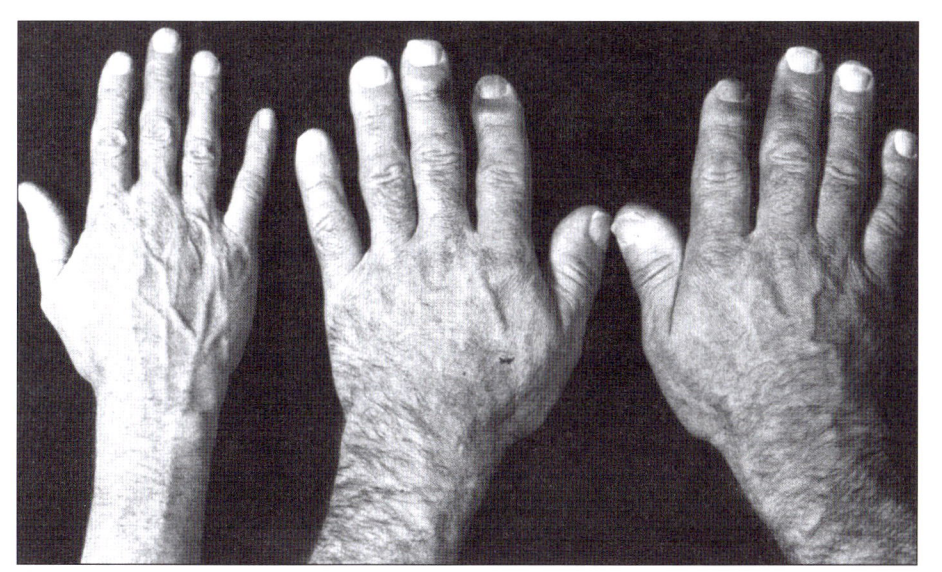

▲ **Figure 2.1** Hand of a normal patient (left) and the hands of a patient with acromegaly (centre and right).

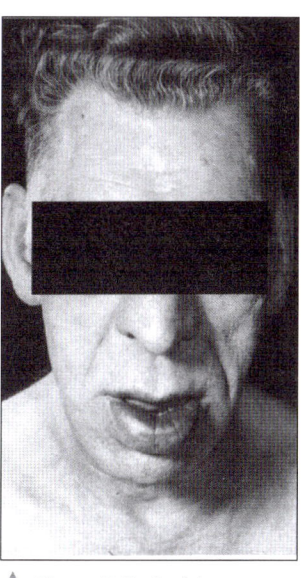

▲ **Figure 2.2** Facial appearance of patient with acromegaly.

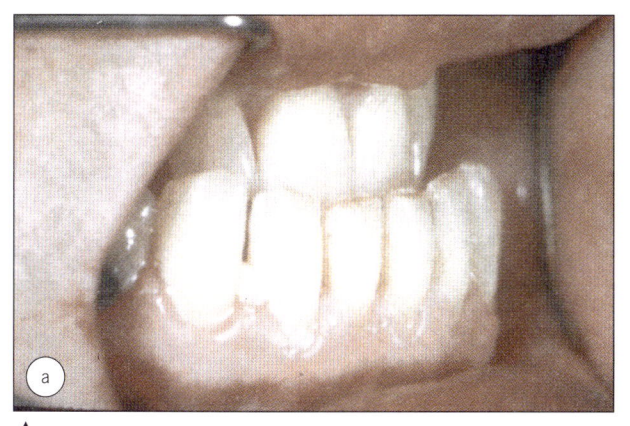

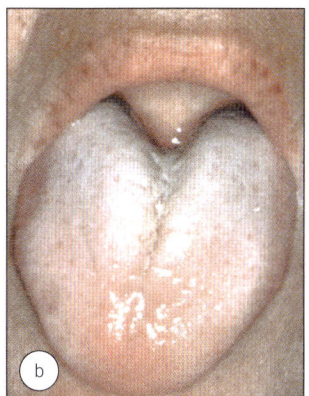

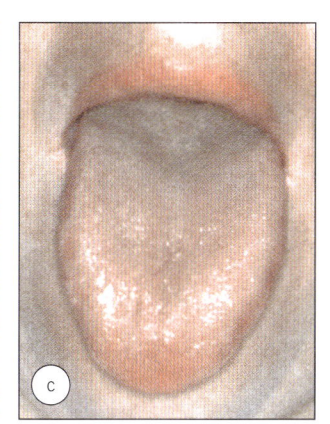

▲ **Figure 2.3** (a) Increased interdentate spacing and prognathism, (b) macroglossia in a patient with acromegaly and (c) a normal tongue.

GH levels. Skin tags and acanthosis nigricans may also be noted.

Cardiac features

Cardiac disease is common in patients with acromegaly, being present in at least one-third of cases at presentation, and it is a major cause of mortality for these patients. Cardiac enlargement is a very common finding, associated with myocardial hypertrophy with interstitial fibrosis, increased left ventricular mass and concentric hypertrophy (Colao et al. 1997). Subsequent ventricular wall dilation and/or ventricular dilatation occurs and leads to biventricular failure. A specific acromegalic cardiomyopathy has been suggested, which can be improved by lowering GH concentrations (Colao et al. 1997).

In addition to structural changes in the heart, the incidence of cardiovascular disease is increased, including coronary artery disease and arrhythmias. Resting electrocardiograms (ECGs) are abnormal in up to 50% of patients with evidence of ischaemia and rhythm and/or conduction disturbance. This is the result of hypertension and impaired glucose tolerance.

Hypertension

Hypertension occurs in approximately one-third of patients at presentation. Aldosterone and plasma renin levels are usually suppressed, and total body sodium is increased. This may arise from a direct effect of GH on sodium transport, with hypertension resulting at least partly from sodium retention and expanded plasma volume. In addition, the effects of acromegaly on left ventricle muscle mass may play a role. Hypertension tends to improve with treatment of acromegaly, although it often does not resolve fully.

Carbohydrate intolerance

Excess GH concentrations lead to insulin resistance in 80% of patients with acromegaly, with impaired glucose tolerance occurring in approximately 40% and diabetes mellitus in 10–25% (Duncan and Wass 1999). These parameters improve with treatment, and complete resolution of diabetes mellitus occurs in two-thirds of patients following successful surgery.

Respiratory disease

Retrospective cohort studies demonstrate that part of the increased mortality in acromegaly results from respiratory disease. Lung size is increased and upper airway obstruction is common in up to 75% of males and 25% of females. This is caused by macroglossia, deformities in the jaw, goitre and epiglottis hypertrophy, and may lead to significant difficulty in intubation.

Obstructive sleep apnoea is common, found in approximately 60% of patients, but it is more common in males than females. Although the majority of cases of sleep apnoea are obstructive, a proportion are central in origin. Treatment of acromegaly may correct sleep apnoea, but some cases may require long-term respiratory support.

Thickening of the vocal cords and enlargement of the sinuses lead to a deep voice.

Malignancy

The majority of retrospective cohort studies demonstrate increased mortality rates for malignancy (Orme et al. 1998, Wright et al. 1970), although this has not been the experience of all investigators (Nabarro 1987). The possible role of paracrine and/or autocrine GH and IGF-I in tumour development in patients without acromegaly and the association between higher IGF-I levels and risk of malignancy (such as prostate and breast cancer in population studies) has increased interest in the possible mechanisms involved. It is likely that the improved treatment of acromegaly (leading to longer life expectancy) is revealing the increased risk of malignancy which may not have been obvious in earlier studies.

The majority of a large number of retrospective studies to investigate the association between acromegaly and colonic malignancy show an increased risk of both benign polyps and malignant tumours (Klein et al. 1982, Ezzat et al. 1991, Ron et al. 1991). More recently a large prospective colonoscopic screening study demonstrated an increased risk of both premalignant and frankly neoplastic colonic tumours (Jenkins et al. 1997). The relationship between GH and IGF-I and the risk of colonic neoplasia is unclear; some studies show no relationship (Jenkins et al. 1997), while others suggest an increased risk with elevated GH concentrations (Orme et al. 1998). On the basis of these studies, the current recommendations for patients with acromegaly are a screening full colonoscopy every 3 years after the age of 40 years.

A possible increase in other tumours, such as breast, thyroid and prostate cancer, has also been suggested. Although the evidence for an increased risk of goitre development and of prostate overgrowth in patients with acromegaly is good, fewer data are available on cancers. Information from large databases and further prospective studies should help to answer these remaining questions.

Bone, joints and neuromuscular disorders

Joint stiffness may be an early feature because of increased subcutaneous tissue, but is reversible on lowering GH concentrations. Up to 75% of patients develop arthropathy, which leads to a destructive osteoarthritis of the weight-bearing joints and is irreversible once established. Carpal tunnel syndrome is present in 35–50% of patients at diagnosis (Molitch 1992). Approximately half the patients have evidence of a proximal myopathy at diagnosis, which improves as GH concentrations are lowered. Bones may be osteopenic because of hypogonadism and hypercalciuric as a result of hypervitaminosis D (see below).

In addition to increased joint space because of soft-tissue enlargement, there may be thickening of the metacarpals, metatarsals, phalanges and articular cartilages. Tufting of the terminal phalanges may be seen on radiography.

Other endocrine dysfunction

Multinodular goitre is common, but hyperthyroidism is found in a minority of cases only. When present hyperthyroidism may worsen cardiac abnormalities. Coexistent TSH secretion from the pituitary adenoma should always be considered if TSH is detectable or elevated in the presence of hyperthyroidism.

Hypercalciuria is common, as GH stimulates 1-α-hydroxylase, leading to increased 1,25-dihydroxycholecalciferol, increased gastric calcium absorption and hypercalciuria. Renal stones occur in up to 10% of cases. In patients with hypercalcaemia, hyperparathyroidism associated with MEN 1 should be considered (3% of patients).

INVESTIGATIONS

Acromegaly is defined biochemically as excessive disordered autonomous secretion of GH. The aim of investigation is to:
- demonstrate excessive GH secretion;
- demonstrate the source of the autonomous secretion (e.g. pituitary micro- or macroadenoma);
- assess the remaining pituitary function, looking for deficiency of trophic hormone secretion and excess PRL secretion; and
- assess the metabolic and structural complications of acromegaly which need intervention.

Biochemical diagnosis of acromegaly

Oral glucose tolerance test

Oral glucose tolerance test (OGTT) is the usual first investigation (*Box 2.2*). In acromegaly, there is failure to suppress GH to <2 mU/l (<1 μg/l) in response to a 75 g oral glucose load. There may even be a paradoxical rise in GH. In addition, OGTT may demonstrate glucose intolerance or frank diabetes mellitus. In contrast, the normal response is GH suppression to undetectable levels.

False positives are given by chronic renal and liver failure, malnutrition, uncontrolled diabetes mellitus, heroin addiction and adolescence.

Box 2.2 Procedure for oral glucose tolerance test

- Patient is fasted from midnight.
- Intravenous cannula is inserted (repeated venepuncture can lead to increase in GH as a stress response).
- At 0900 h (time 0) 75 g glucose is administered.
- Samples for GH and glucose are collected at 30 min intervals from −30 to 150 min.

Random or basal GH

Random or basal GH is not useful in the diagnosis of acromegaly as, although normal healthy subjects have undetectable GH levels throughout the day, there are pulses of GH that are impossible to differentiate from the levels seen in acromegaly. False positives may occur, as shown in *Box 2.3*.

Box 2.3 Differential diagnosis of elevated growth hormone

- Pain
- Pregnancy
- Puberty
- Stress
- Chronic renal failure
- Heart failure
- Diabetes mellitus
- Malnutrition
- Prolonged fast

Insulin-like growth factor-I

In addition to OGTT, IGF-I is useful in differentiating patients with acromegaly from those without, as it is almost invariably elevated in acromegaly except in severe intercurrent illness. As IGF-I is bound to binding proteins it has a long half-life, and reflects the effect of GH on tissues. Many investigators suggest that this is an appropriate cost-effective initial screening test for acromegaly. However, abnormalities of GH secretion may remain while IGF-I is normal.

IGF binding protein-3

IGF binding protein-3 (IGFBP3) concentrations correlate with IGF-I, and some investigators have advocated the use of this assay in both the diagnosis and monitoring of acromegaly. However, although some studies show no overlap between newly diagnosed patients and normal controls, others show that there is overlap. The assay for IGFBP3 is not as widely available as GH and IGF-I. Its role in investigation remains to be fully established, but it may be helpful to measure IGFBP3 in borderline cases because increased IGFBP3 levels have been shown in patients with glucose-suppressible GH and only minimally elevated IGF-I.

Urinary GH

The pulsatile pattern of GH makes the potential use of 24 hour or overnight urinary GH assessment an attractive idea. Data suggest a good correlation between urinary GH and serum GH, IGF-I and activity of acromegaly. Further information is required on the reliability of assays. However, this may become a useful screening test or monitor of disease activity.

GH-releasing hormone

Occasionally it is not possible to demonstrate a pituitary tumour, or pituitary histology reveals hyperplasia. A serum GHRH in addition to radiology of the chest and abdomen may then be indicated to identify the cause.

Inferior petrosal sinus sampling (IPSS) for GH concentrations has been used to lateralise a microadenoma that is not visible on magnetic resonance imaging (MRI) or to demonstrate lack of lateralisation in suspected somatotroph hyperplasia. The combination of IPSS and administration of exogenous GHRH may provide additional information.

Thyrotrophin-releasing hormone test

A paradoxical rise (by 50% over basal, or an increment of at least 10 mU/l (5 µg/l)) in GH following the administration of thyrotrophin-releasing hormone (TRH, Box 2.4) is a characteristic of 50–80% of patients with acromegaly, whereas normal controls do not show a GH response.

This test is usually not required, as the OGTT and IGF-I tests usually provide the diagnosis. It may be helpful in patients with equivocal results.

Box 2.4 Procedure for thyrotrophin-releasing hormone test

- Patient is fasted from midnight.
- Intravenous cannula is inserted (repeated venepuncture can lead to increase in GH as stress response).
- At 0900 h (time 0) 200 µg TRH is administered intravenously.
- Samples for GH and TSH are collected at 30 min intervals from –30 to 120 min.

Dopaminergic tests

Dopaminergic substances lead to a rise in GH in normal subjects, but in 50–80% of patients with acromegaly there may be a paradoxical fall in GH (Box 2.5).

Box 2.5 Procedure for dopamine test

- Patient is fasted from midnight.
- Two intravenous cannulae are inserted.
- At 0900 h (time 0) dopamine is infused at 4 µg/ml (8 mU/l) per min for 3 h.
- Samples for GH measurement are collected at 30 min intervals from –30 min to 2 h after the infusion was stopped.

Alternative
- Oral bromocriptine 2.5 mg at time 0.
- Monitor GH at time 0 and hourly for 6 h.

GH day curve

Measurements of GH are taken at 4–5 time points during the day. This is used to assess cure following surgery or radiotherapy, and also to assess GH suppression on somatostatin analogues to determine whether an increase in dose is required. It does not have a role in the diagnosis of acromegaly.

Determination of cause of acromegaly

Usually MRI demonstrates the tumour, the presence of extrasellar extension and whether this is suprasellar or into the cavernous sinus (Fig. 2.4). In addition, plain radiographs may demonstrate enlargement of the pituitary fossa and frontal sinuses, although these are usually not performed routinely.

It is important, particularly in the case of macroadenomas, to document visual acuity formally

CLINICAL FEATURES, INVESTIGATION AND COMPLICATIONS OF ACROMEGALY

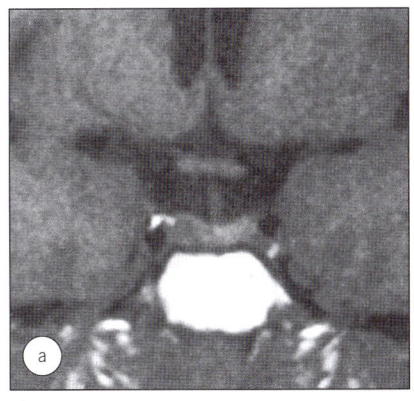

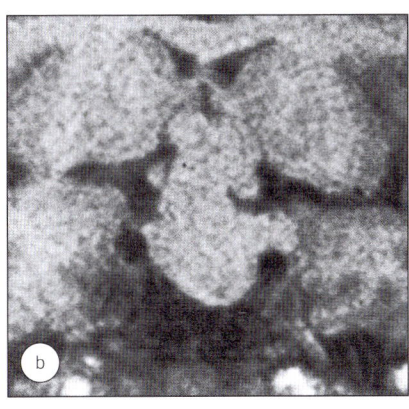

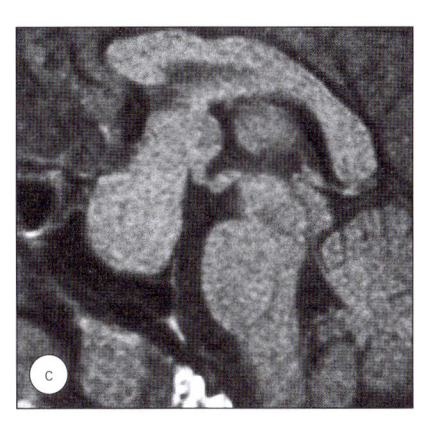

Figure 2.4 Magnetic resonance imaging scans of pituitary tumours causing acromegaly. (a) Coronal section showing right-sided microadenoma. (b) Coronal section showing large invasive macroadenoma extending into the cavernous sinus and suprasellar region. (c) Sagittal section showing macroadenoma with suprasellar extension.

and to map the visual fields with Goldmann perimetry (or similar).

Somatostatin receptor scintigraphy

Conflicting data exist on the use of this mode of imaging. Administration of a radiolabelled somatostatin analogue has been used to detect occult tumours and to predict the response to therapy using somatostatin analogues. The density of receptors and labelling technique influence the results and more data are required on the use of this imaging mode.

Assessment of residual pituitary function

Serum PRL should be measured as some tumours cosecrete both GH and PRL. The gonadotrophin, TSH and ACTH axes should be assessed using basal hormonal concentrations and, where necessary (e.g. ACTH reserve), a stimulation test.

Assessment of complications of acromegaly

Table 2.5 shows the metabolic and structural complications of acromegaly that need intervention and their assessment.

ASSESSMENT OF COMPLICATIONS OF ACROMEGALY

System	Disorder	Investigation	Management
Cardiac	Left ventricular hypertrophy, dilatation and cardiac failure Ischaemic heart disease Arrhythmias	Echocardiography (ECG) Resting ECG ± exercise testing 24 h ECG monitoring	Optimise cardiac risk factors, e.g. hypertension diabetes, smoking, hyperlipidaemia
Hypertension		24 h monitoring may be helpful	Treatment – ?target for therapy <140/80 mmHg
Carbohydrate intolerance	Impaired glucose tolerance Diabetes mellitus	Fasting glucose and insulin HbA1c	Diet ± tablet ± insulin therapy Modification of associated metabolic risk factors, e.g. hyperlipidaemia and hypertension
Respiratory disease	Obstructive sleep apnoea	Sleep studies	Ventilatory support, e.g. nocturnal continuous positive airways pressure
Calcium and bone	Hypercalciuria Hypercalcaemia (?primary hyperparathyroidism) Osteopenia	Serum and urinary calcium Parathyroid hormone Bone mineral density	Renal ultrasound may be required if stones are suspected Consider antiresorptive therapy
Malignancy	?Colon ??Breast	Colonoscopy every 3 years after age 40 years or if suggestive symptoms, and more frequently if polyps detected Vigilance for features suggesting other tumours	

Table 2.5 Assessment of complications of acromegaly.

References

Asa SL & Kovacs K 1992 Pituitary pathology in acromegaly. *Endocrinology and Metabolism Clinics of North America* **21** 553–574.

Bates AS, Van'T Hoff W, Jones JM & Clayton RN 1993 An audit of outcome of treatment in acromegaly. *Quarterly Journal of Medicine* **86** 293–299.

Bertherat J, Chanson P & Montminy M 1995 The cyclic adenosine 3´,5´-monophosphate-responsive factor CREB is constitutively activated in human somatotroph adenomas. *Molecular Endocrinology* **9** 777–783.

Colao A, Merola B, Ferone D & Lombardini G 1997 Extensive personal experience of acromegaly. *Journal of Clinical Endocrinology and Metabolism* **82** 2777–2781.

Duncan E & Wass JAH 1999 Investigation protocol: acromegaly and its investigation. *Clinical Endocrinology (Oxford)* **50** 285–293.

Ezzat S, Strom C & Melmed S 1991 Colon polyps in acromegaly. *Annals of Internal Medicine* **114** 754–755.

Jenkins PJ, Fairclough PD, Richards T et al. 1997 Acromegaly, colonic polyps and carcinoma. *Clinical Endocrinology (Oxford)* **47** 17–22.

Klein I, Parveen G, Gavoeler JS & Van Thiel DH 1982 Colonic polyps in patients with acromegaly. *Annals of Internal Medicine* **97** 27–30.

Molitch M 1992 Clinical manifestations of acromegaly. *Endocrinology and Metabolism Clinics of North America* **21** 597–614.

Nabarro JDN 1987 Acromegaly. *Clinical Endocrinology* **26** 481–512.

Orme SM, McNally RJQ, Cartwright RA & Belchetz PE 1998 Mortality and cancer incidence in acromegaly: A retrospective cohort study. *Journal of Clinical Endocrinology and Metabolism* **83** 2730–2734.

Rajasoorya C, Holdaway IM, Wrightson P, Scott DJ & Ibbertson HK 1994 Determinants of clinical outcome and survival in acromegaly. *Clinical Endocrinology* **41** 95–102.

Ron E, Gridley G, Hrubec Z, Page W, Arora S & Fraumeni JF Jr 1991 Acromegaly and gastrointestinal cancer. *Cancer* **68** 1673–1677.

Swearingen B, Barker FG, Katznelson L et al. 1998 Long-term mortality after trans-sphenoidal surgery and adjunctive therapy for acromegaly. *Journal of Clinical Endocrinology and Metabolism* **83** 3419–3426.

Wright AD, Hill DM, Lowy C & Fraser TR 1970 Mortality in acromegaly. *Quarterly Journal of Medicine* **34** 1–16.

Zhang X, Horwitz GA, Heaney AP et al. 1970 Pituitary tumour transforming gene expression in pituitary adenomas. *Journal of Clinical Endocrinology and Metabolism* **84** 7611–767.

3

THE AIMS OF TREATMENT AND DEFINITION OF CURE FOR ACROMEGALY

3 THE AIMS OF TREATMENT AND DEFINITION OF CURE FOR ACROMEGALY

John Wass Department of Endocrinology, Radcliffe Infirmary, Oxford, UK

INTRODUCTION

The aims of treatment of acromegaly have been clear for many years. Regrettably, it is equally clear that over 100 years after the original description of the disease, these aims are all achievable in only a very small minority of the patients treated. This applies to all modalities of treatment currently available, whether applied together, as they are for some patients, or singularly in an individual patient.

In contrast to the clarity of the aims of treatment of acromegaly, which have not changed, the definition of cure in acromegaly has changed over the years and continues to do so. As short a period of time ago as 1998 it was clear that a glucose tolerance test (GTT) nadir of growth hormone (GH) <2 µg/l (4 mU/l) was the definition (Melmed et al. 1998). Very recently this criterion has become more stringent and cure is now defined as a GTT nadir GH <1 µg/l (2 mU/l; Giustina et al. 2000). It is likely that in the future the biochemical diagnosis of cure will become even more restricted, in part because of improved and more sensitive assays for GH (as discussed below).

The definition of cure and the criteria used make an enormous difference to the percentages achieved in different series. Earlier surgical data quoted GH levels <10 µg/l (20 mU/l) as cure. Current epidemiological data show that normal mortality is associated with a mean ambient GH level of 5 mU/l, but some investigators use a GTT nadir GH of 2.0 µg/l. There is a high correlation of 99% between these two values (Ahmed et al. 1999). In the Osman series from Newcastle (Osman et al. 1994) a GTT nadir GH <2 mU/l (<1 µg/l) was achieved in 48.6%, a mean GH of 5 mU/l (2.5 µg/l) in 59.2%, a minimum GH after a GTT of 5 mU/l (2.5 µg/l) in 76.3% and a basal GH of <20 mU/l (<10 µg/l) in 90.8% of cases. Such differences in assessing the results of various series make it essential that the criteria used to define cure are carefully noted as they make a major difference to the outcome percentages. Nowadays, for the moment at least, the internationally agreed criteria (Giustina et al. 2000) should be used.

One other general point is important, namely that 'cure' is a frequently used term in the acromegalic literature. In fact it is very uncommon to achieve a complete biochemical cure with a normal GH suppression after an oral GTT, and undetectable GH levels for the majority of the day with the normal pulsatility of GH. It is therefore probably more accurate not to refer to different GH levels as 'cure', but to describe GH levels that are safe (i.e. not associated with an increased mortality).

AIMS OF TREATMENT

The aims of treatment of acromegaly are shown in *Table 3.1*. They are discussed individually below and an attempt is made to describe how the different modalities, namely transsphenoidal surgery, medical treatment and radiotherapy, attain these.

Relief of symptoms
Complete symptomatic relief of acromegaly is not always attained, even if GH levels are completely

THE AIMS OF TREATMENT OF ACROMEGALY
Relief of symptoms
GH secretion normal
Reversal of somatic changes and metabolic abnormalities – diabetes mellitus, hypercalciuria
Ablate tumour mass
No recurrence of tumour
Minimum disturbance to patient
No side effects, e.g. hypopituitarism
No mortality
Achieve normal life expectancy

▲ Table 3.1 The aims of treatment of acromegaly.

normalised (for symptoms of acromegaly, see *Table 2.4*). As GH levels fall there is marked improvement, initially in soft-tissue changes. As GH causes salt and water retention, when GH levels suddenly become normal from being considerably elevated, particularly postoperatively, a marked diuresis can occur, often confused with diabetes insipidus. Excessive sweating stops with the attainment of normal GH levels and the symptoms of carpal tunnel compression reverse. However, excessively high blood pressure does not always become normal, though it usually improves, and cardiomyopathy, if it has developed, may improve, but more frequently does not revert to normal.

A major debate is taking place on the problem of colonic polyps in acromegaly, but the general view is that the frequency of colonic polyps and colon cancer is increased in acromegaly. If present and treated, the available data suggest that these polyps are less likely to recur in patients with GH levels that have been rendered normal by various treatments than in those patients with persistently active acromegaly.

Osteoarthritis, particularly in the knees and hips, is a problem in acromegaly that does not reverse with successful treatment. This is a cogent argument for diagnosing acromegaly early.

Reversibility of somatic changes

This is often quick if the somatic changes are mild. Soft-tissue changes occur first, as noted above, but bony changes may take months or even years to reverse. In patients with advanced disease the bony changes may never completely reverse. It is clear that acromegaly is diagnosed earlier nowadays than it was in the 1930s, so now more frequently than not somatic and bony changes eventually reverse; of course, this happens most quickly in those patients with mild disease.

With regard to the different modalities of treatment for the relief of symptoms and the reversibility of somatic changes, this is quickest in patients after successful surgery or after drug treatment that renders normal either both GH and insulin-like growth factor-I (IGF-I) or just IGF-I in the case of GH-receptor antagonists. The relief of symptoms and the reversal of somatic changes are much slower after radiotherapy, the effects of which can continue to reduce GH and IGF-I for over 15 years.

The attainment of normal growth hormone levels

In normal subjects GH is undetectable for the majority of the day apart from peaks that occur intermittently during the day itself and more frequently during the

AIMS OF TREATMENT MATCHED TO DIFFERENT AVAILABLE METHODS IN ACROMEGALY

Symptom	Surgery		Drugs			Radiotherapy		Comments
	Micro-adenoma	Macro-adenoma	Somatostatin analogues	Dopamine agonists	GH-receptor antagonists	External beam	Gamma knife	
Relief of symptoms	+++	++	++	+	+++	+	++	
GH secretion/ IGF-I 'normal' or 'safe'	90%	50%	50–80%	20%	>90%	@ 10 years GH 60%, IGF-1 55%	?	IGF-1 only for pegvisomant GH levels remain high
Recurrence of tumour	5–7%	5–7%				Very uncommon		
Hypopitu-itarism	10–20%	10–20%	Does not occur			At 10 years very common		Gonadotrophins 80%, adrenocorticotrophic hormone 20%, thyroid-stimulating hormone 60% (Jenkins *et al.* 2000)
Mortality	Occasional	Occasional	Does not occur	Does not occur		Does not occur		

▲ **Table 3.2** Aims of treatment matched to different available methods in acromegaly.

night. After an oral GTT the GH value falls to below 0.5 mU/l (0.25 µg/l) and the GH-dependent growth factor IGF-I is normal for the age of the patient (it has different normal ranges at different ages). It is rare to achieve normality in all of these modalities (*Table 3.2*).

After surgery, in good surgical hands, safe GH values should be achieved with microadenomas in around 90% and with macroadenomas in over 50% of cases. However, rates vary and only the best tend to be reported (Osman *et al*. 1994, Abosch *et al*. 1998, Swearingen *et al*. 1998, Ahmed *et al*. 1999). The UK Acromegaly Database provides evidence of this, and analysis of the results from various centres that have no dedicated pituitary surgeon shows outcome figures that are much less good (e.g. microadenomas 'cured' in 38% (Lissett *et al*. 1998) as opposed to 90% of cases. Clearly, as well as tumour size, surgical experience is important (Clayton *et al*. 1999, Turner & Wass 2000).

With regard to drugs the outcome is more reproducible. Currently, long-acting release octreotide (octreotide-LAR) and slow-release lanreotide (lanreotide-SR) are most used. Overall around 50% of patients in unselected series obtain normal GH and IGF-I values. However, in some series, particularly those in which the initial GH is low, higher numbers of cases, around 80%, can achieve normal IGF-I values (Turner *et al*. 1999). Using dopamine agonists, either cabergoline or bromocriptine, around 20% of patients obtain a normal GH or IGF-I. With pegvisomant, the new GH-receptor antagonist, which is currently unavailable, data suggest that normal IGF-I values can be obtained in over 90% of patients. GH levels do not change (Trainer *et al*. 2000).

The effects of external beam radiotherapy on GH and IGF-I levels take much longer to achieve. The maximum response is in the first 2 years, during which an exponential decline in GH occurs. By 10 years around 60% of patients have GH levels <2.5 µg/l and 55% of patients have a normal IGF-I (Jenkins *et al*. 2000). Other data (Powell *et al*. 2000) suggest roughly similar figures with normal IGF-I values at 6 years in 69% and GH values below 2.5 µg/l in 44% of cases. It is clear from studies of GH levels throughout 24 hours in patients who have had acromegaly that GH pulsatility is completely abolished by external beam radiotherapy (Peacey *et al*. 1998).

Further data are required to establish whether the gamma knife achieves normal GH levels more quickly than ordinary external beam radiotherapy.

Reversible metabolic abnormalities

The frequency with which diabetes occurs in association with acromegaly is around 30%, but the actual figure depends on the definition of diabetes used. With any treatment modality blood glucose levels fall towards normal, but glucose tolerance does not always become normal, particularly in long-standing acromegalic patients (Wass *et al*. 1980). Thus, after surgery carbohydrate tolerance can be expected to improve, particularly if normal GH levels are obtained. Using octreotide or lanreotide, despite the suppression of insulin, which is of much shorter duration than that of GH, carbohydrate tolerance improves. Currently no data reported in the literature show the effect of pegvisomant on carbohydrate tolerance.

Another (but less important) metabolic effect of high GH levels is that of hypercalciuria, because GH is facultative in the synthesis of vitamin D and levels of 1,25-dihydroxyvitamin D_3 are elevated in acromegaly. Thus, 80% of patients with acromegaly have hypercalciuria and there is a small increase in incidence of renal calculi in patients with acromegaly (5%). No studies show whether or not this reverses, but the expectation is that with the attainment of normal GH all therapies would render increased calcium excretion normal.

Ablation of tumour mass

With surgery the aim is self-evidently to ablate the tumour. This is usually achievable in patients with microadenomas, but not always in those with macroadenomas. Young patients particularly tend to have very large extrasellar tumours that behave aggressively and in some cases even transcranial surgery may not achieve ablation completely. It is clear that the vast majority of patients with acromegaly can be treated surgically by the transsphenoidal route, and only very rarely is the transcranial one necessary.

Medical treatment does not have a major effect on tumour mass. With the somatostatin analogues, decreases in tumour size are observed in about 40% of cases, but these reductions are relatively minor, particularly compared with the considerable changes that can occur with the treatment of prolactinomas by dopamine agonists. No significant benefit has been shown from the decrease in size of GH-secreting pituitary tumours induced by somatostatin analogues. Similarly, the dopamine agonists cabergoline and bromocriptine induce small decreases in tumour size in patients treated successfully. Again no clinical benefit from this change has been shown. With pegvisomant no change has been shown in the size of the majority of tumours, but two tumours increased slightly in size with this drug. The majority of the data currently in the literature describe patients treated with radiotherapy, so it is important to obtain further data on the effect of pegvisomant on tumour size in patients untreated with radiotherapy. Currently, the data do not show any trend toward an increase in tumour size.

Radiotherapy on its own has little effect on tumour size. It is often given after incomplete surgery, at which time GH levels are persistently elevated.

Recurrence of tumour

After surgery the incidence of recurrence is low, from 5 to 7%. Usually these recurrences are mild, but they may occur at any time up to 15 years after the initial surgery. Recurrence seems less common than in patients with Cushing's disease. Similarly, untreated nonfunctioning tumours recur at a much higher rate (50% at 10 years). Interestingly, our surgeon in Oxford adopts a more aggressive surgical approach to patients with Cushing's disease than to those with acromegaly, but nevertheless our recurrence rate in patients with Cushing's disease is higher (Yap et al. 2001). Clearly, in Cushing's and acromegaly we are dealing with two different disease processes.

Tumour enlargement has not been described after drug therapy with octreotide, lanreotide or dopamine agonists. As described above, it has rarely been described with pegvisomant but more data are needed.

With radiotherapy tumour control is obtained in the vast majority of patients, and regrowth of tumours after radiotherapy is very uncommon indeed (<5%).

Patient disturbance

As shown in Table 3.1, one of the aims of treatment is to minimise the disturbance to patients. In this respect, the variation between the different modes of treatment is substantial.

For surgery, patients are admitted for between 3 and 7 days. After transsphenoidal surgery nasal packs can be uncomfortable for a short period of time, but the patients very rapidly make a good recovery and, unless side effects occur, there are no long-term sequelae.

Octreotide-LAR is administrable every 28 days, and maybe it can be administered less frequently. Lanreotide is administrable every 7–21 days. Both are given by intramuscular injection, which can often be carried out by local practice nurses with a minimum of effort. Pegvisomant is administrable as a daily injection. Dopamine agonists are administrable orally, but of course are effective less often.

Radiotherapy is a major undertaking that requires careful planning and daily visits for 5 weeks to a radiotherapy department that has experience in pituitary radiotherapy. Radiotherapy to the pituitary can be administered once only, except in very exceptional circumstances.

Side effects
Hypopituitarism

Surgery causes new hypopituitarism in between 10 and 20% of patients according to the series. New gonadotrophin deficiency occurs most frequently, followed by new adrenocorticotrophic hormone (ACTH) deficiency and then thyroid-stimulating hormone (TSH) deficiency. In good surgical hands it is also possible to improve function, and in the Oxford series (Ahmed et al. 1999) pituitary function improved in over 30% of patients. Deteriorating pituitary function occurs with all sizes of tumour to the same extent.

Somatostatin analogues, dopamine agonists and GH-receptor antagonists do not cause any change in pituitary function.

Radiotherapy causes a time-dependent deterioration in pituitary function, such that at 10 years nearly 80% of patients are gonadotrophin deficient with 20% ACTH deficient and 60% TSH deficient. Radiotherapy given to a patient for acromegaly makes it imperative that regular pituitary function tests are carried out every year or every other year.

Surgery

The complication rate seems to vary quite widely from 4 to 18%. It is not clear whether this results from the use of different diagnostic criteria or because complication rates vary with different surgeons. Certainly, in the Oxford series (Ahmed et al. 1999) complication rates did not vary with surgical experience and time, whereas overall success did; it is clear that the outcome in terms of GH levels postoperatively improved over time. Surgical complications include diabetes insipidus (1–7%), cerebrospinal fluid leak, meningitis and haemorrhage.

Drugs

The side effects of octreotide and lanreotide are given in Table 3.3. Dopamine agonists also cause side effects, particularly at the initiation of treatment; these include nausea, vomiting and postural hypotension. The longer term side effects include constipation, a Raynaud-like phenomenon in some

SIDE EFFECTS OF SOMATOSTATIN ANALOGUES IN THE TREATMENT OF ACROMEGALY

Type	Description
Local	Stinging at the injection site (warm prior to injection)

Gastrointestinal	Short term:
	  diarrhoea
	  abdominal pain
	Long term:
	  gall stones
	  gastritis

Biochemical	Antibody formation
Endocrinological	Worsening carbohydrate tolerance Hypoglycaemia
Dependency	

Table 3.3 Side effects of somatostatin analogues in the treatment of acromegaly.

patients and, in others on very high dosages, hypomania and sleeplessness.

Pegvisomant may very occasionally cause abnormalities of liver function.

Radiotherapy

Besides hypopituitarism, radiotherapy is associated with hair loss at the site of entry of the three portals. This is reversible. Using the currently widely accepted prescription of 4500 cGy over 25 days at 180 cGy per day, visual disturbances have been reported in fewer than 10 patients worldwide. There is a suggestion in the literature that visual damage is more common in patients who are elderly, hypertensive and in whom radiotherapy is given to tumours in contact with the with optic chiasm. Cases are too few to be certain, but in our practice we avoid radiotherapy before the chiasm is properly decompressed surgically (Jones 1991).

Some data suggest an increase in the number of second malignancies after radiotherapy. At 10 years Brada *et al.* (1992) report a second malignancy rate of 2%. Another series (Jones 1991) does not report second malignancy. It seems possible that the rate of second malignancy in the field of radiotherapy is increased, but the numbers are small and the data inconclusive.

Lastly, another suggestion in the literature, which is currently unproved, is that mental changes and memory loss occur after pituitary radiotherapy. No adequate studies have been published to document this or conclude that it is not a phenomenon.

Mortality

Most surgical series report no mortality. Anaesthesia in severe acromegaly can be difficult and respiratory complications can occur. However, the vast majority of surgical series report no mortality perioperatively.

Self-evidently, drugs and radiotherapy are not associated with any mortality.

Life expectancy

The aim of treatment is to produce a normal life expectancy in patients with acromegaly. Mortality is at least doubled in untreated acromegaly (Wright *et al.* 1970). Successful treatment should be associated with a normal life expectancy compared to the normal population. What has not been clear until recently is the GH and IGF-I criteria that are associated with a normal life expectancy; upon these criteria rests the definition of 'cure' or what exactly is meant by 'safe' GH levels.

DEFINITION OF CURE OF ACROMEGALY

The currently accepted definition of cure is shown in *Table 3.4*. In reality this is not 'cure'. After surgery it is often the case that GH levels remain detectable, whereas in normal subjects they are undetectable, and that after surgery pulses are not normal in frequency or size. After radiotherapy pulsatility is lost too. Despite this a number of series (Bates *et al.* 1993, Orme *et al.* 1998) show that if GH levels of 2.5 µg/l (5 mU/l) or below are obtained the mortality is the same as that for the normal population. The Bates study reported small numbers only, but in the Orme study the same findings were confirmed in larger numbers. Thus it seems that a basal random or a mean of several GH values of 2.5 µg/l (5 mU/l) is associated with a normal mortality and that this should be an aim of treatment.

With regard to the response to oral GTT, this should fall to <1 µg/l (<2 mU/l). While few epidemiological studies have examined this specific

DEFINITION OF CURE OF ACROMEGALY

Test	Criterion
Random or mean GH	<2.5 µg/l (<5 mU/l)
Oral glucose tolerance test GH nadir	<1.0 µg/l (<2 mU/l)
Normal age-related IGF-I	

Table 3.4 Definition of cure of acromegaly.

criterion, there is a very good correlation (99%) between a basal GH of 2.5 µg/l (5 mU/l) and a nadir GH of 1 µg/l (2 mU/l) during an oral GTT (Osman et al. 1994, Ahmed et al. 1999). It is therefore safe to conclude that this is an alternative or an additional criterion for safe GH levels, albeit not absolutely normal.

Only one series so far has looked at IGF-I values as outcome criteria (Swearingen et al. 1998). This series had IGF-I data for the majority of patients and concluded that a normal IGF-I was associated with a normal mortality. More data on IGF-I are needed, in particular because of the discordance between normal IGF-I values and GH data in a minority of patients. Nevertheless, for a successful outcome of treatment, IGF-I should be within the age-related normal range. For those patients in whom it was not, there was a 3.5% increase in relative mortality risk (Swearingen et al. 1998).

Growth hormone assays

The above discussions do not take into account the different GH assays utilised throughout the world. Until fairly recently, polyclonal radioimmunoassays were used in the majority of laboratories. These assays are much less sensitive than the more modern immunoradiometric assays, which better differentiate normality from unsuccessfully treated acromegaly (Freda et al. 1998). It is possible that when highly sensitive enzyme-linked immunoabsorbent assays become widely available the diagnostic criteria will change further with the necessity to attain even lower GH levels. Clearly, for the correct interpretation of GH results it is essential for endocrinologists to know which GH assay is being used by the laboratory.

Modality of treatment and their individual effects

The above discussion on the attainment of normal life expectancy with treatment does not discuss individual modalities of treatment in relation to life expectancy. The available data relate to the attainment of GH values by several different means including surgery, radiotherapy and drugs. As yet no data suggest that one or other modality of treatment favours the attainment of a normal life expectancy. The early suggestions are that in some cases the administration of radiotherapy predisposes to cerebral vascular morbidity and even mortality, but further data from larger numbers of patients are necessary.

CONCLUSIONS

The aims of treatment are clear, but we remain unable to attain them in all but a minority of patients with acromegaly. The current definition of cure is clear and as endocrinologists we should audit our results, including surgical results, in relation to these (Giustina et al. 2000).

References

Abosch A, Tyrrell JB, Lambrown KR, Hannegan LT, Applebury CB & Wilson CB 1998 Transsphenoidal microsurgery for growth hormone secreting pituitary adenomas: initial outcome and long-term results. *Journal of Clinical Endocrinology and Metabolism* **83** 3411–3418.

Ahmed S, Elsheikh M, Page RCL, Adams CBT & Wass JAH 1999 Outcome of transsphenoidal surgery for acromegaly and its relationship to surgical experience. *Clinical Endocrinology* **50** 561–567.

Bates AS, Van't Hoff W, Jones JM & Clayton RN 1993 An audit of outcome of treatment in acromegaly. *Quarterly Journal of Medicine* **86** 293–299.

Brada M, Ford D, & Ashley S 1992 Risk of second brain tumour after conservative surgery and radiotherapy for pituitary adenoma. *British Medical Journal* **304** 1343–1346.

Clayton RN, Stewart PM, Shalet SM & Wass JAH 1999 Pituitary surgery for acromegaly: the case for many fewer surgeons. *British Medical Journal* **319** 588–589.

Freda PU, Post KD, Powell JS & Wardlaw SL 1998 Evaluation of disease status with sensitive measures of growth hormone secretion in 60 postoperative patients with acromegaly. *Journal of Clinical Endocrinology and Metabolism* **83** 3808–3816.

Giustina A, Barkan A, Casanueva FF et al. 2000 Criteria for cure of acromegaly: a consensus statement. *Journal of Clinical Endocrinology and Metabolism* **85** 526–529.

Jenkins PJ, Elliot EL & Carson MM 2000 The effects of pituitary irradiation on serum GH and IGF-I levels in acromegaly – results from the UK National Database. Abstract 2163 from the Endocrine Society's 82nd Annual Meeting.

Jones A 1991 Radiation oncogenesis in relation to the treatment of pituitary tumours. *Clinical Endocrinology* **35** 379–397.

Lissett CA, Peacey SR, Laing I, Tetlow L, Davis JRE & Shalet SM 1998 The outcome of surgery for acromegaly: the need for a specialist pituitary surgeon for all types of growth hormone secreting adenoma. *Clinical Endocrinology* **49** 653–657

Melmed S, Jackson I, Kleinberg D & Klibanski A 1998 Current treatment guidelines for acromegaly. *Journal of Clinical Endocrinology and Metabolism* **83** 2646–2652.

Orme SM, McNally RJQ, Cartwright RA & Belchetz PE 1998 Mortality and cancer incidence in acromegaly: a retrospective cohort study. *Journal of Clinical Endocrinology and Metabolism* **83** 2730–2733.

Osman IA, James RA, Chatterjee K, Mathias D & Kendall-Taylor P 1994 Factors determining the long-term outcome of surgery for acromegaly. *Quarterly Journal of Medicine* **87** 617–623.

Peacey SR, Toogood AA & Shalet SM 1998 Hypothalamic dysfunction in 'cured' acromegaly is treatment modality dependent. *Journal of Clinical Endocrinology and Metabolism* **83** 1682–1686.

Powell JS, Wardlaw SL, Post KD & Freda PU 2000 Outcome of radiotherapy for acromegaly using normalisation of insulin-like growth factor I to define cure. *Journal of Clinical Endocrinology and Metabolism* **85** 2068–2071.

Swearingen B, Barker FG, Katznelson L et al. 1998 Long-term mortality after transsphenoidal surgery and adjunctive therapy for acromegaly. *Journal of Clinical Endocrinology and Metabolism* **83** 3419–3426.

Trainer PJ, Drake WM, Katznelson L et al. 2000 Treatment of acromegaly with the growth hormone receptor antagonist pegvisomant. *New England Journal of Medicine* **342** 1171–1177.

Turner HE, Vadivale A, Keenan J & Wass JAH 1999 A comparison of lanreotide and octreotide LAR for treatment of acromegaly. *Clinical Endocrinology* **51** 275–280.

Turner HE & Wass JAH 2000 Modern approaches to treating acromegaly. *Quarterly Journal of Medicine* **93** 1–6.

Wass JAH, Cudworth AG, Bottazzo GF, Woodrow JC & Besser GM 1980 An assessment of glucose intolerance in acromegaly and its response to medical treatment. *Clinical Endocrinology* **12** 53–59.

Wright AD, Hill DM, Lowy C & Fraser TR 1970 Mortality in acromegaly. *Quarterly Journal of Medicine* **34** 1–16.

Yap LB, Adams CBT, Turner HE & Wass JAH 2001 Undetectable post-operative cortisol does not always predict long term remission in Cushing's disease, even in good surgical hands. *Clinical Endocrinology* in press.

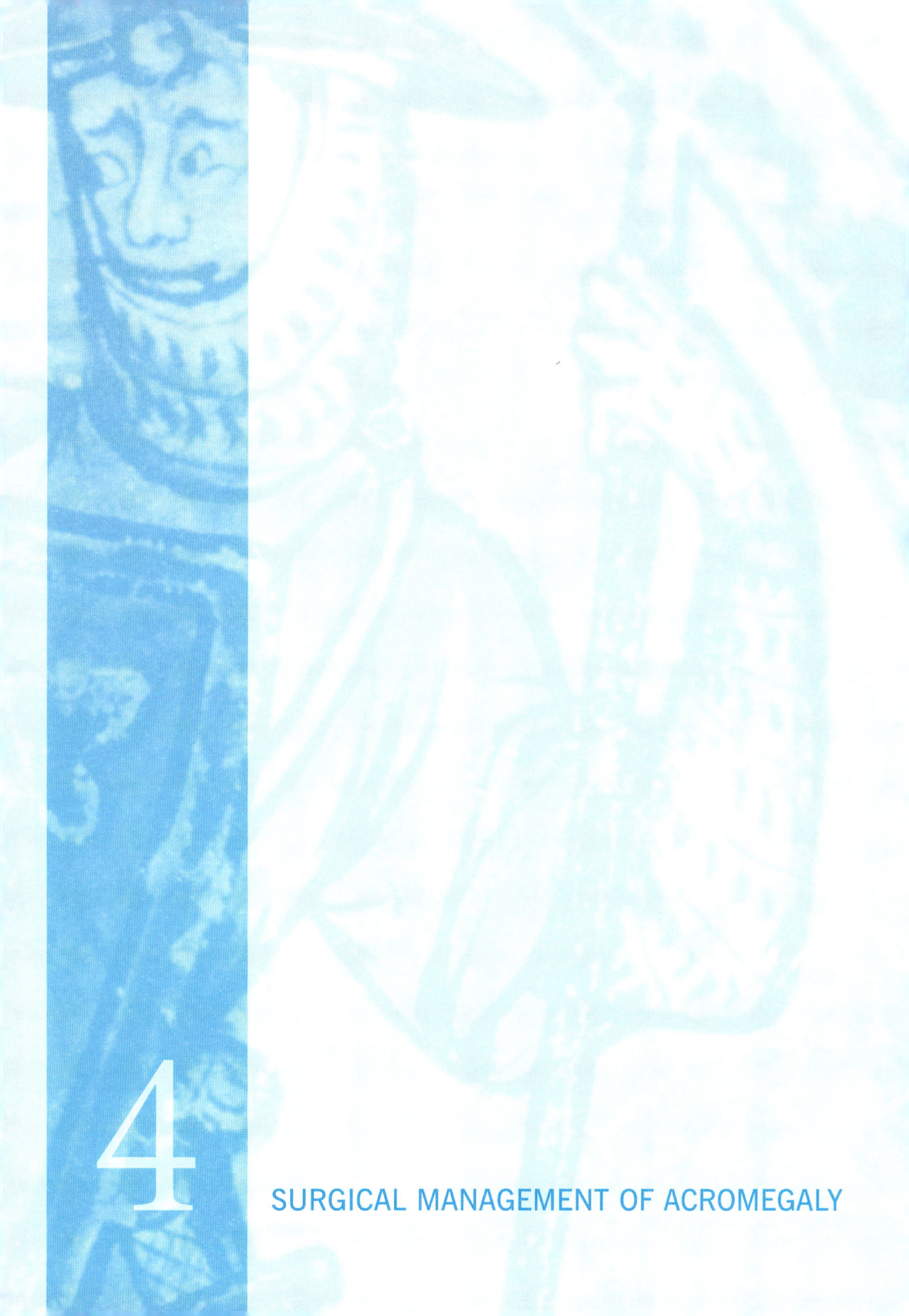

4

SURGICAL MANAGEMENT OF ACROMEGALY

4 SURGICAL MANAGEMENT OF ACROMEGALY

Rudolph Fahlbusch, Michael Buchfelder, Jürgen Kreutzer and Panos Nomikos Department of Neurosurgery, University of Erlangen–Nürnberg, Erlangen, Germany

INTRODUCTION

Acromegaly is a serious disease and studies suggest that mortality in acromegaly is approximately double that in the general population. The cause of death is most commonly vascular, but significant increases have been reported for deaths from both respiratory disorders and malignancies. Therefore, aggressive management to lower serum growth hormone (GH) levels is necessary once the diagnosis has been confirmed. For the majority of patients the first-line therapy is surgery, either alone or in conjunction with radiotherapy and/or medical therapy. In this chapter we report on the surgical results of a consecutive series of acromegalic patients treated in the Department of Neurosurgery at the University of Erlangen–Nürnberg and also summarise the experiences of other surgeons most commonly reported in the literature. Other treatment options, such as medical therapy and radiotherapy are discussed in other chapters of this book.

PATIENT SERIES

In the past 17 years (December 1982 to January 2000), 640 operations (490 primary and 150 secondary surgery) for GH-secreting pituitary adenomas have been performed in our department. Of these, 583 patients presented with signs and symptoms of acromegaly and 12 with gigantism. There were 317 females and 278 males (ratio female:male = 1.14:1.0).

ENDOCRINOLOGICAL EVALUATION

Preoperatively, basal fasting levels of GH, insulin-like growth factor I (IGF-I; determined routinely since 1989), prolactin, cortisol, gonadotrophins, testosterone, oestradiol, thyroid-stimulating hormone, free thyroxine and free tri-iodothyronine were measured in the serum of all patients. In every case an oral glucose tolerance test (OGTT) was performed. Pituitary stimulation as a combination of adrenocorticotrophin (ACTH), thyrotrophin-releasing (TRH) and luteinising hormone-releasing hormone (LHRH) tests or the ACTH test alone was used to reveal preoperative partial deficiencies of the anterior lobe of the pituitary. The same tests were repeated 7 days and 3 months after surgery. These results were analysed to estimate the remission rates. Follow-up examinations were held mostly at annual or biannual visits. However, several patients referred from abroad were lost to follow up.

Reviewing published series shows considerable confusion in the literature as to what should be regarded as the biochemical definition of cure (*Box 4.1*). In most early published reports of surgical results, a single basal GH level below 5 or even 10 µg/l (10 or 20 mU/l) is used to confirm a surgical success. We consider this definition inadequate, since the episodically secreted GH levels fluctuate widely and many of these patients later present with 'recurrent' acromegaly. For our series, surgical success is best defined by normalisation of the basal GH level below 5 µg/l (10 mU/l), suppression of GH to <2 µg/l (<4 mU/l) during OGTT and normal IGF-I (definition 1 in *Box 4.1*). With these values, no clinical signs of acromegaly were found and recurrence was exceptionally rare. This condition also correlated excellently with the improvement or regression of diabetes mellitus and arterial hypertension in a considerable number of patients. In our study, remission was achieved if all three criteria were fulfilled during the endocrinological follow-up 3 months after surgery. We have also analysed the data according to the most recent definition of cure (definition 2 in *Box 4.1*), as described by Giustina *et al.* (2000). Throughout the text remission rates are given according to definition 2, with the equivalent figure for definition 1 following in brackets.

Box 4.1 Definitions of cure

Definition 1
- Normalisation of the basal GH level below 5 μg/l (10 mU/l)
- Suppression of GH to <2 μg/l (<4 mU/l) during OGTT
- Normal IGF-I

Definition 2
- Normalisation of the basal GH level below 2.5 μg/l (5 mU/l)
- Suppression of GH to <1 μg/l (<2 mU/l) during OGTT
- Normal IGF-I

SURGICAL TREATMENT

The vast majority of the operations (n = 621) were performed by the transsphenoidal route. In 18 cases with invasive, asymmetrical suprasellar, retrosellar and/or supraclinoidal parasellar extension, transcranial surgery via a pterional approach was used and only in one case (with an invasive adenoma in the interhemispheric region) was a bifrontal approach required. Combined transsphenoidal and transcranial approaches were used to treat 14 patients.

For the transsphenoidal approach, the patient's positioning and principles originally described by Harvey Cushing were used: the patient is positioned supine with the head tilted downwards about 10° and the surgeon standing behind the patient's head (*Fig. 4.1*). A unilateral paraseptal approach was used most often, with a mucosal incision usually made in the vestibulum nasi along the cartilaginous nasal septum. Alternatively, a sublabial incision was used. The mucosa and both the nasal cartilaginous and bony septum are usually hypertrophied in acromegaly, making the approach difficult in many cases. A Cushing-type speculum was inserted and the mostly thickened floor of the sphenoid sinus opened using a diamond drill under the microscope. The whole sella turcica from the sphenoidal plane to the clivus was exposed and the sellar floor then opened and completely resected to the medial wall of the cavernous sinus. The basal dura was opened. A small biopsy was taken to rule out tumour invasion histologically. The tumour was removed using various curettes and microforceps. In case of cerebrospinal fluid (CSF) leak, the sellar floor was sealed with two pieces of muscle fascia from the lateral thigh fixed by fibrin glue. A lumbar drainage was placed for CSF drainage until

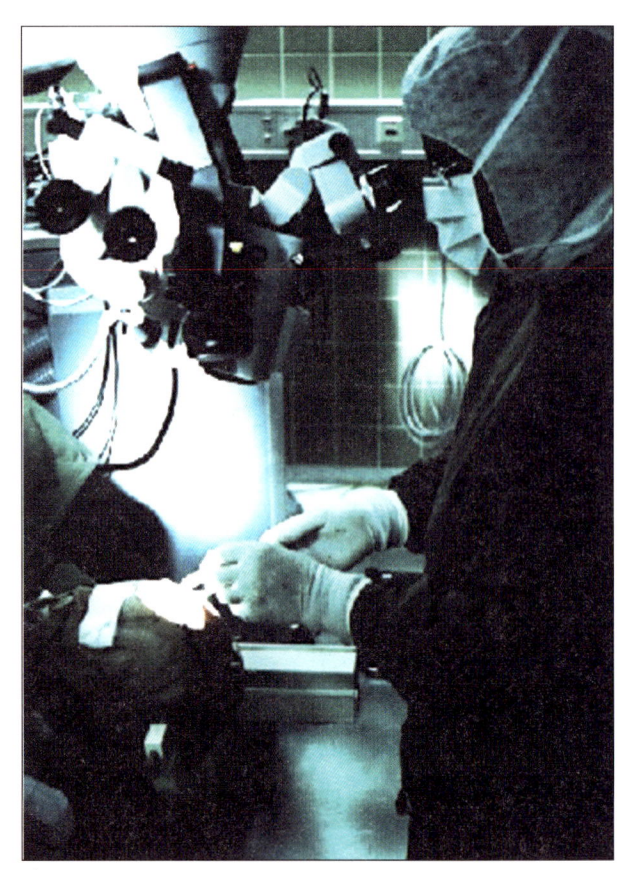

▲ **Figure 4.1** Even when the surgeon uses modern equipment like neuronavigation and endoscopy, the standard transsphenoidal approach with the surgeon standing behind the patient's head, as first described by Harvey Cushing, is still used in our department.

the third postoperative day. The mucosal incision was then closed and both tamponades inserted into both nostrils for 24 h. Technical variations, such as the use of the endoscope or the direct approach through the nasal cavity, are discussed later.

The transcranial approach should be avoided in acromegaly since craniotomy may be very difficult because of major ossification of the frontal bone and large frontal sinuses. If not avoidable, in our series a small standard pterional craniotomy was usually used. The tumour was resected piecemeal by incising the tumour capsule and performing an intracapsular reduction of tumour tissue. The capsule was then mobilised, preserving the perforating arteries to the hypothalamic region and the optic nerves. With respect to tumours invading the cavernous sinus, the increasing amount of resectable tumour mass was accompanied by a higher morbidity, particularly of optomotor nerve dysfunction. Despite extensive manipulations, total tumour resection and normalisation of GH hypersecretion are not usually achieved by surgery alone in these cases.

MORTALITY AND MORBIDITY

Mortality was fortunately rare: only one patient (0.15%), who had a giant adenoma, died after transsphenoidal surgery. Morbidity was very low: meningitis and CSF leaks occurred in <1% of cases. The complication rate in repeat transsphenoidal surgery was not significantly different from that found in primary procedures.

RESULTS

Depending on the growth characteristics, degree and direction of extrasellar expansion, GH-secreting adenomas were classified as microadenomas (tumour diameter ≤ 10 mm), macroadenomas (tumour diameter 11–39 mm) and giant adenomas (tumour diameter ≥ 40 mm). Macroadenomas were further divided into intrasellar tumours (IS), parasellar and/or sphenoidal tumours (PS/SPHE), suprasellar tumours without visual compromise (S1) and suprasellar tumours with visual compromise (S2).

An overview of the remission rates in the different categories following primary transsphenoidal surgery is provided in *Table 4.1*, which gives the results according to both definitions of cure in *Box 4.1*. The overall rate of endocrinological remission was 53% (56%) with 27% of the tumours having an invasive character (*Fig. 4.2*). Invasion was recognised either intraoperatively or during histological work-up. The best results were achieved in the microadenoma and

REMISSION RATES FOLLOWING PRIMARY TRANSSPHENOIDAL SURGERY

Tumour extension		Remission rate (%)	
		Definition 1 (basal GH <5 µg/l (<10 mU/l), OGTT GH <2 µg/l (<4 mU/l), normal IGF-I)	Definition 2 (basal GH <2.5 µg/l (<5 mU/l), OGTT GH <1 µg/l (<2 mU/l), normal IGF-I)
Microadenomas		78	72
Macroadenomas	Intrasellar	78	74
	Parasellar and/or sphenoidal	44	40
	Suprasellar without visual compromise	48	44
	Suprasellar with visual compromise	37	33
Giant adenomas		0	0
All adenomas		56	53

Table 4.1 An overview of the remission rate in the different categories of tumours following primary transsphenoidal surgery (n = 490) and respecting different criteria for biochemical cure: 27% of the tumours were found to be invasive.

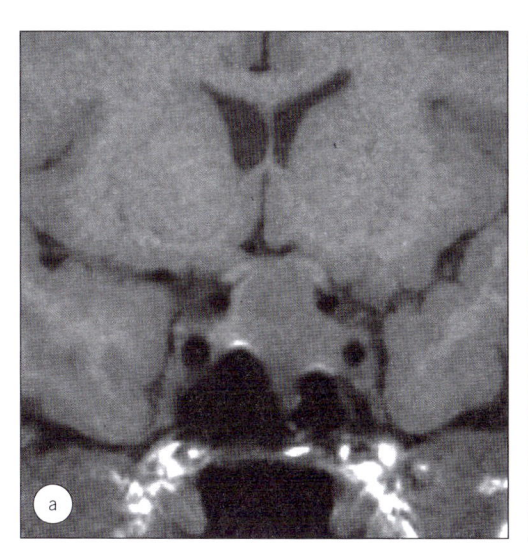

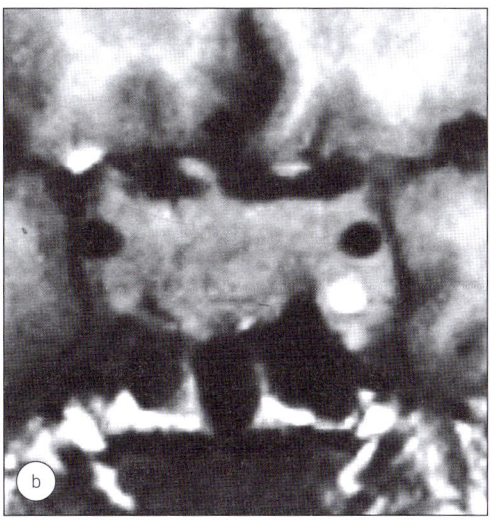

Figure 4.2 Invasive GH-secreting adenomas. (a) Invasion into the sphenoid sinus. In these cases the invasive part of the tumour can be completely resected together with a portion of the sella floor. (b) Parasellar invasion into the cavernous sinus. In such cases endocrinological remission by surgery alone is not possible.

IS macroadenoma groups with 72% and 74% (78% and 78%), respectively, considering all three criteria for biochemical cure. Remission rates tended to drop in the more extensive macroadenomas: 44% (48%) for S1 and 33% (37%) for S2 and 40% (44%) for tumours with PS/SPHE expansion. In giant adenomas, only in one case was biochemical cure achieved by surgery alone.

Transcranial surgery was performed mostly for invasive asymmetrical lesions that extended into the suprasellar area or as a combined approach before or after transsphenoidal surgery. In line with the characteristics of these lesions, the overall remission rate was only 5.26% (15.7%). The transcranial group consisted of S2 macroadenomas and giant adenomas, which were usually very extensive and frequently had an invasive character. Transcranial surgery yielded remission rates of 7.69% (23%) and 0%, respectively.

Surgical re-exploration was usually carried out for noninvasive adenomas not cured by primary surgery. Re-explorations of the sella were considered particularly when the magnetic resonance images (MRIs) clearly demonstrated residual adenoma tissue. Such reoperations were performed in 150 cases in this series. In this group the overall remission rate was 21.3% (28.5%). Another indication for repeat surgery was reduction of the tumour mass in surgically not totally resectable adenomas to establish better conditions for further medical and radiation treatment.

DISCUSSION

The goals of surgical therapy in acromegaly include:
- initial endocrinological remission with normalisation of the dynamic GH-secretion pattern as well as normalisation of basal IGF-I to give regression of the signs and symptoms of the disease;
- prevention of recurrence (long-term remission) and
- performance of selective adenomectomy (preservation of normal pituitary functions).

As a result of the difficulties in defining postoperative endocrinological remission and the variations in criteria used by different investigators (Giustina et al. 2000), the success rates in terms of achievement of these goals vary significantly in the published series from different institutions (Table 4.2).

In early series, the criterion for remission was a postoperative GH-level below 5 µg/l (10 mU/l). Ross and Wilson in 1988 analysed the results of 30 published series and yielded an overall 'cure' rate of 56% in 153 cases. In another multicentre study published in 1987 by Zervas the overall 'cure' rate was 66% in 1256 cases. Using the GH response after an oral glucose load to assess the effectiveness of surgery, rates of endocrinological remission were found to be lower, as in our previous series (Fahlbusch et al. 1992). In this series, the remission rate was 71% with a basal GH level below 5 µg/l (10 mU/l) as the criterion, but

PRIMARY TRANSSPHENOIDAL SURGERY FOR GH-SECRETING PITUITARY ADENOMAS

Series	Number of cases	Total cure rate (%)	Microadenomas (%)	Macroadenomas (%)	Definition of 'cure'
Ross and Wilson 1988	153	56	N/A	N/A	GH <5 µg/l (<10 mU/l)
Losa et al. 1989	29	55	N/A	N/A	GH <1 µg/l (<2 mU/l) and normal IGF-I levels
Fahlbusch et al. 1992	222	57	72	49	GH <2 µg/l (<4 mU/l) OGTT
		71	81	65	GH <5 µg/l (<10 mU/l)
Tindall et al. 1993	91	82	N/A	N/A	GH <5 µg/l (<10 mU/l) and/or normal IGF-I levels
Davis et al. 1993	174	52	N/A	N/A	GH ≤2 µg/l (<4 mU/l; basal or OGTT)
Sheaves et al. 1996	100	42	61	23	GH ≤2.5 µg/l (<5 mU/l)
Abosch et al. 1998	254	76	75	71	GH <5 µg/l (<10 mU/l)
Freda et al. 1998	115	61	88	53	GH <2 µg/l (<4 mU/l) OGTT or normal IGF-I levels
Ahmed et al. 1999	97	–	90	56	Basal GH ≤2.5 µg/l (≤5 mU/l), OGTT GH ≤1 µg/l (≤2 mU/l), normal IGF-I levels
Laws et al. 2000	117	67	87	50.5	Basal GH ≤2.5 µg/l (≤5 mU/l), OGTT GH ≤1 µg/l (≤2 mU/l), normal IGF-I levels
This series	490	56	78	50	Basal GH ≤5 µg/l (≤10 mU/l), OGTT GH ≤2 µg/l (≤4 mU/l), normal IGF-I levels

▲ Table 4.2 Results of primary transsphenoidal surgery for GH-secreting pituitary adenomas.

this dropped significantly to 57% with a glucose-suppressed GH level below 2 µg/l (4 mU/l) as the criterion for endocrinological remission. Similar results were found in other series published by Losa et al. (1989) and Valdemarsson et al. (1991). The use of all three criteria, including normalisation of basal IGF-I, does not further change the previously reported endocrinological remission rates, as shown by Tindall et al. (1993) and Laws et al. (2000).

Similar results were found in this current series. The overall rate for endocrinological remission with respect to normalisation of basal GH (below 5 µg/l (10 mU/l)), to normalisation of IGF-I and to GH-levels below 2 µg/l (4 mU/l) during OGTT was found to vary between 36 and 82% (using the stricter criteria of definition 2 changes these figures only modestly). Several factors could be detected as predictors of the surgical result, such as tumour size, invasiveness, extrasellar growth, and secretory activity.

Regarding the growth characteristics of the lesions, microadenomas have a more favourable surgical outcome than macroadenomas, particularly those with extrasellar extension. In microadenomas, a remission rate as high as 82% could be achieved. With increasing tumour diameter and extrasellar extension, remission drops stepwise to 0% for giant adenomas. Similar results are found in other published series, as in the outcome analysis of Tindall et al. (1993) and Ross and Wilson (1988). The main reason for this drop is the increasing number of invasive growth patterns in larger adenomas. Pituitary adenomas are considered invasive if they have infiltrated or perforated the normal anatomical confines of the pituitary gland, namely the sellar diaphragm, basal dura, clivus or sphenoidal and cavernous sinuses. Although invasion tends to be more common with increasing tumour size, microadenomas may also have an invasive character and conversely large tumours may reach a considerable size simply by displacing the adjacent anatomical structures without actually invading them.

Localised or generalised invasion, however, should not be equated with malignancy of the tumour. The diagnosis of pituitary carcinoma is only exceptionally justified when subarachnoid dissemination, brain or distant metastases are documented. No carcinomas were observed in this study. Invasion can be documented by intraoperative findings, neuroradiological investigations and/or histological examination. Surgical invasion describes the invasive nature of the tumour as recognised during operation, while histological invasion, although more frequent, can only be demonstrated by investigating the anatomical structures in the vicinity of the tumour. In up to 80% of cases dural invasion is detected when the basal dura is thoroughly investigated (Ahmadi et al. 1986, Buchfelder et al. 1996). In this series, the overall remission rate of noninvasive adenomas was 76% and dropped to 24% for invasive tumours (using definition 1 for cure). Also, for transcranial surgery increased invasiveness of the tumour is the main reason for incomplete tumour resection and persistent disease.

The secretory activity of the adenoma also influences the response to surgical therapy, as observed in several published series (Ross and Wilson 1988, Tindall et al. 1993, Sheaves et al. 1996). Various thresholds of preoperative basal GH levels between 40 and 70 µg/l (80 and 140 mU/l) have been proposed. Preoperative GH levels above these values have an inverse relationship with the likelihood of biochemical remission following surgery. In our previously published series (Fahlbusch et al. 1992), we observed that this inverse relationship has an almost linear character. In the present series, this linear relationship is confirmed. If a basal GH level of 50 µg/l (100 mU/l) is defined as an arbitrary threshold for the secretory activity of an adenoma, then the overall cure (definition 1) rate drops from 74% in cases with preoperative GH levels below this threshold to 25% in cases with preoperative GH levels above it.

The frequency of tumour recurrence is strongly associated with the remission criteria used. It is paramount to distinguish between postoperative normalisation of GH secretion using all three criteria (in definition 1) and those cases with lower postoperative basal levels of GH but an inadequate response to OGTT and/or abnormal IGF-I levels. Using a postoperative basal GH below 5 µg/l (10 mU/l) as the remission criterion, the overall 'recurrence' rate in 61 patients was 7% over a mean follow-up period of 6 years (Fahlbusch et al. 1992). Similar results were published by Arafah et al. (1987) and Losa et al. (1989). However, using suppression of GH levels below 2.5 µg/l (5 mU/l) as the criterion, long-term remission can be achieved, as observed by our group (Buchfelder et al. 1991), although in other published series rates of recurrence up to 17.8% (Davis et al. 1993) are encountered with other criteria for biochemical cure. In the present series, a mean follow-up period of more than 10 years (10.7) has been observed. During this period and using all three criteria (in definition 1) for biochemical cure, only four patients (about 1%) with recurrent acromegaly presented 3–6 years after initial surgery. This fact stresses the paramount importance of stringent endocrinological remission criteria in acromegaly.

The management of patients with persistent acromegaly after the first operation is a matter of ongoing discussion. Several meetings have been held to obtain a consensus as to how these patients should be treated ideally. All treatment modalities concerning this disease have been discussed in detail. We strongly feel that many of these patients are candidates for repeat surgery. Re-exploration was found to be particularly successful for those patients in whom neither surgical nor histological invasion could be demonstrated during the first surgery. In this series, re-explorations were performed in 150 cases, mainly for patients with MRI studies that demonstrated residual adenomatous tissue. The overall remission rate was, of course, worse than in the primary surgery group, at 21.3% (28.5%). Nevertheless, a remission rate of 37.3% (48%) could be achieved in patients with noninvasive tumours and an initial GH level below 40 µg/l (80 mU/l) prior to the first surgical approach. The absence of both major surgical complications and any significant endocrinological deterioration of other pituitary functions supports re-exploration as a treatment option in a number of patients with persistent acromegaly.

The results in this series, once more, strongly support the role of surgery as the primary management option for acromegalic patients. Surgery is very efficacious in restoring normal GH secretion patterns, acts rapidly and carries a low therapy-associated morbidity. From the economic point of view, surgery is less expensive than long-term medical treatment with GH-suppressing drugs. Furthermore, patients who meet strictly defined endocrinological remission criteria have an excellent long-term prognosis and for this reason (expensive) follow-up examinations are required only sporadically. It is also clear that surgical experience, skill and knowledge play an important role in how successful the primary surgery is (Lisett et al. 1998, Ahmed et al. 1999). The results presented in this chapter concern only those series published by authors with major expertise in this field and cannot be achieved by surgeons with little experience in pituitary surgery. Supraregional specialisation in a few neurosurgical centres with equally experienced endocrinologists and laboratory staff may lead to even better surgical results in acromegaly.

Only recently, new surgical techniques that utilise new technical possibilities have been applied (Fahlbusch et al. 1996, Fahlbusch 1999). The use of an endoscope, with its major advantage of panoramic visualisation of the anatomical structures through the wide angle of view and powerful light devices, makes the extended transsphenoidal approach to parasellar lesions safer (Fig. 4.3). Additionally, the direct nasal approach, which avoids paraseptal preparation, renders postoperative nasal tamponades no longer necessary

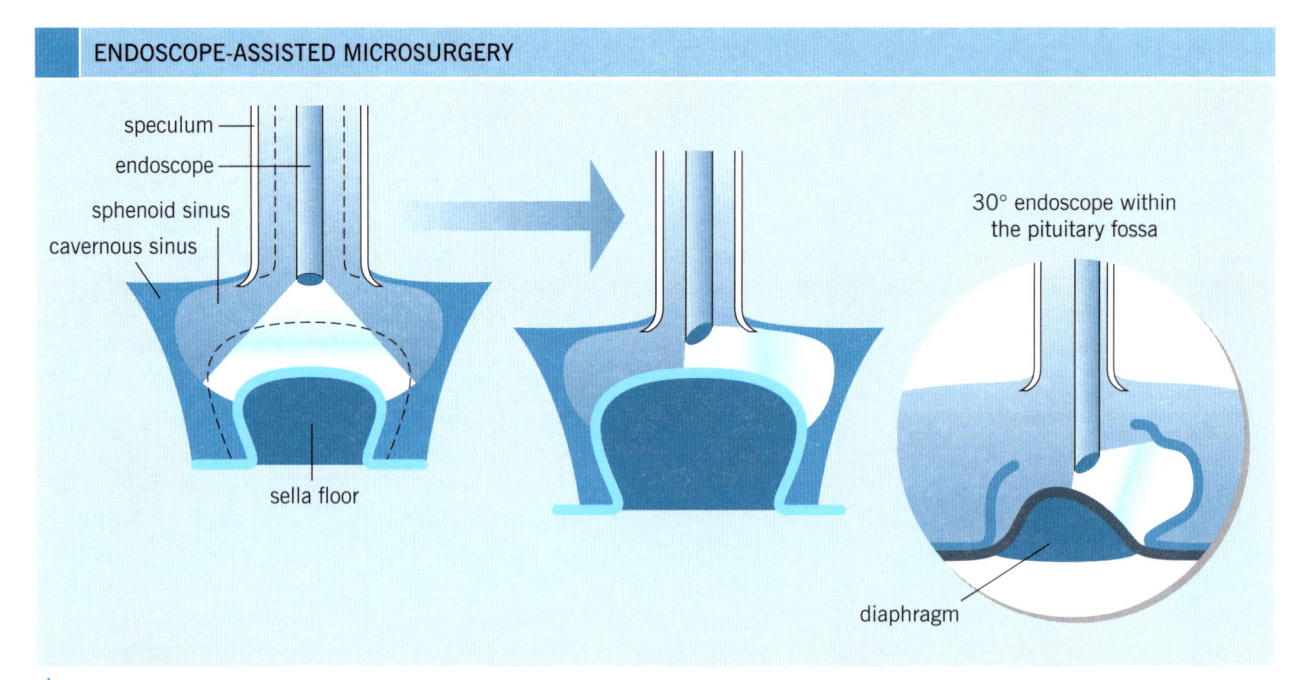

▲ **Figure 4.3** Endoscope-assisted microsurgery involves the standard equipment of transsphenoidal surgery supported by an endoscope, which provides a panoramic view of the sphenoid sinus. Using a 30° endoscope a view 'around the corner' is possible. Parasellar structures can be visualised and any residual tumour detected and resected.

and therefore leads to a better subjective feeling for the patient because of free nasal ventilation. Indeed, for such patients hospitalisation of 1 day only has been suggested. Neuronavigation is helpful for the localisation of anatomic structures intraoperatively. This method allows virtual surgery with segmentation and three-dimensional reconstruction of the tumour and its adjacent structures by superimposing the tumour margins and the carotid arteries, and therefore allows a safe approach to the sella even in cases with narrow sellar floors and loss of anatomical landmarks in reoperations. Intraoperative MRI, until recently only available in a few centres, allows neurosurgeons to perform surgery interactively using MRI guidance and, more importantly, allows intraoperative resection control in large intra- and parasellar tumours. However, the extent to which these technical advances will improve the endocrinological results of surgery in acromegalic patients needs to be investigated further.

References

Abosch A, Tyrrell JB, Lamborn KR, Hannegan LT, Applebury CB & Wilson CB 1998 Transsphenoidal microsurgery for growth hormone-secreting pituitary adenomas: initial outcome and long-term results. *Journal of Clinical Endocrinology and Metabolism* **83** 3411–3418.

Ahmed S, Elsheikh M, Stratton IM, Page RCL, Adams CBT & Wass JAH 1999 Outcome of transsphenoidal surgery for acromegaly and its relationship to surgical experience. *Clinical Endocrinology* **50** 561–567.

Ahmadi J, North CM, Segall HD, Zee CS & Weiss MH 1986 Cavernous sinus invasion by pituitary adenomas. *AJR: American Journal of Roentgenology* **146** 257–262.

Arafah BM, Rosezweig JL, Fenstermaker R et al. 1987 Value of growth hormone dynamics and somatomedin-C (insulin-like growth factor I) levels in predicting the long-term benefit after transsphenoidal surgery for acromegaly. *Journal of Laboratory Clinical Medicine* **109** 346–354.

Buchfelder M, Brockmeier S, Fahlbusch R et al. 1991 Recurrence following transsphenoidal surgery for acromegaly. *Hormone Research* **35** 113–118.

Buchfelder M, Fahlbusch R, Adams EF, Kiesewetter F & Thierauf P 1996 Proliferation parameters for pituitary adenomas. *Acta Neurochirurgica* **65** 18–21.

Davis D, Laws ER Jr, Ilstrup D et al. 1993 Results of surgical treatment for growth hormone-secreting pituitary adenomas. *Journal of Neurosurgery* **79** 70–75.

Fahlbusch R 1999 Future avenues in treatment of pituitary adenomas. *Pituitary* **2** 113–116.

Fahlbusch R, Honegger J & Buchfelder M 1992 Surgical management of acromegaly. *Endocrinology and Metabolism Clinics of North America* **21** 669–692.

Fahlbusch R, Heigl T, Huk WJ et al. 1996 The role of endoscopy and intraoperative MRI in transsphenoidal pituitary surgery. In *Pituitary Adenomas*, pp 237–244. Eds K von Werder & R Fahlbusch. Amsterdam: Excerpta Medica Elsevier.

Freda PU, Wardlaw SL & Post KD 1998 Long-term endocrinological follow-up evaluation in 115 patients who underwent transsphenoidal surgery for acromegaly. *Journal of Neurosurgery* **89** 353–358.

Giustina A, Barkan A, Casanueva FF et al. 2000 Criteria for cure of acromegaly: a consensus statement. *Journal of Clinical Endocrinology and Metabolism* **85** 526–529.

Laws ER, Vance ML & Thapar K 2000 Pituitary surgery for the management of acromegaly. *Hormone Research* **53** (Suppl 3) 71–75.

Lisett CA, Peacey SR, Laing I, Tetlow L, Davis JRE & Shalet SM 1998 The outcome of surgery for acromegaly: the need for a specialist pituitary surgeon for all types of growth hormone (GH) secreting adenomas. *Clinical Endocrinology* **49** 653–657.

Losa M, Oeckler R, Schopohl J et al. 1989 Evaluation of selective transsphenoidal adenomectomy by endocrinological testing and somatostatin-C measurement in acromegaly. *Journal of Neurosurgery* **70** 561–567.

Ross DA & Wilson CB 1988 Results of transsphenoidal microsurgery for growth hormone-secreting pituitary adenomas in a series of 214 patients. *Journal of Neurosurgery* **68** 854–867.

Sheaves R, Jenkins P, Blackburn P et al. 1996 Outcome of transsphenoidal surgery for acromegaly using strict criteria for surgical cure. *Clinical Endocrinology* **45** 407–413.

Tindall G, Oyesiku N, Watts N et al. 1993 Transsphenoidal adenomectomy for growth hormone secreting pituitary adenomas in acromegaly: outcome analysis and determinants of failure. *Journal of Neurosurgery* **78** 205–215.

Valdemarsson S, Bramnert M, Cronquist S et al. 1991 Early postoperative basal serum GH level and the GH response to TRH in relation to the long-term outcome of surgical treatment for acromegaly: a report on 39 patients. *Journal of Internal Medicine* **230** 49–54.

Zervas N 1987 Multicenter surgical results in acromegaly. In *Growth Hormone, Growth Factors, and Acromegaly*, pp 253–257. Eds D Lüdecke & G Tolis. New York: Raven Press.

5

MEDICAL THERAPY

5 MEDICAL THERAPY FOR ACROMEGALY

Aart J van der Lely Department of Internal Medicine, Erasmus University Medical Centre Rotterdam, Rotterdam, Netherlands
Steven Lamberts Department of Medicine, University Hospital of Rotterdam, Netherlands

INTRODUCTION

The treatment of acromegaly has changed considerably during recent decades. In the late 1970s, the introduction of dopamine-receptor agonists made it possible to reduce growth hormone (GH) secretion by somatotropinomas. Thereafter, the introduction of the somatostatin analogues in the early 1980s had major implications for treatment. Recently, data have become available on the use of genetically engineered human GH (hGH) receptor antagonists to block GH action, and so reduce both the biochemical abnormalities of acromegaly and improve clinical signs and symptomatology. In this chapter we give a practical overview of the indications, efficacy and side effects, as well as the place of these three medical treatment modalities.

CURE CRITERIA FOR TREATMENT EVALUATION

According to a recent consensus meeting on the treatment of acromegaly, biochemical control is achieved when all the parameters of disordered GH secretion are restored to normal. Biochemically, this is evident when circulating insulin-like growth factor-I (IGF-I) is reduced to within the age- and sex-adjusted normal range, while nadir GH after an oral glucose load is <1 µg/l (< 2.7 mU/l (Fig. 5.1; Melmed et al. 1998, Giustina et al. 2000)).

SOMATOSTATIN ANALOGUES

Introduction

Some 30 years ago, a hypothalamic factor that regulated GH secretion was discovered accidentally (as reviewed in Lamberts et al. 1996). Later, this somatotroph inhibitory factor was called somatostatin (SST). It is a cyclic peptide of 14 amino acids (SS-14), but there is also a longer form of 28 amino acids (SS-28). A neurotransmitter in the central nervous system, it regulates pituitary GH and thyroid-stimulating hormone (TSH) release as a neurohormone. Also, SST inhibits many physiological actions in different organ systems via autocrine, paracrine and/or neuronal regulation. These different actions of SST are mediated via specific membrane receptors. The presence of SST receptors (SSTRs) has been demonstrated in various regions of the brain, the anterior pituitary, the endocrine and exocrine pancreas, the mucosa of the gastrointestinal tract and in tissues involved in the immune system. Its ability to inhibit many functions of different organs potentially gives SST therapeutic value in clinical conditions that involve hyperfunction of these systems.

Most human tumours originating from SST target tissues show conserved expression of a high density of SSTR. Most GH and TSH-secreting pituitary tumours express SSTR subtypes 2 and 5 (SSTR-2 and -5). No SSTRs have been found on adrenocorticotrophin (ACTH)-secreting pituitary adenomas of patients with Cushing's disease. However, most

CRITERIA FOR CURE OF ACROMEGALY

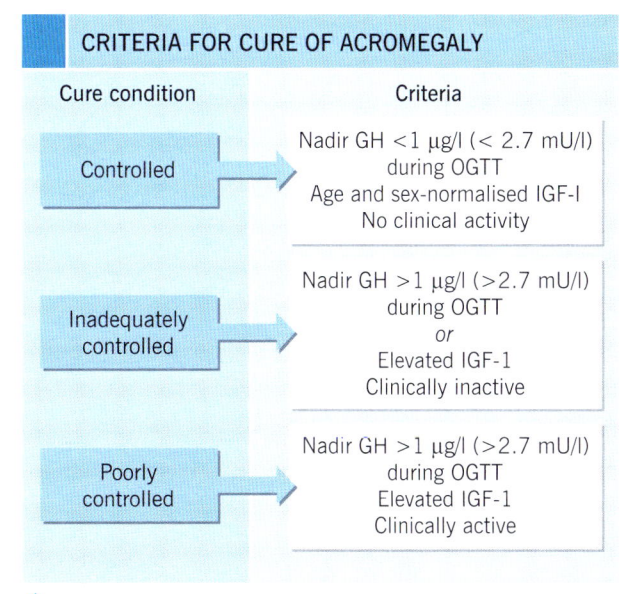

Cure condition	Criteria
Controlled	Nadir GH <1 µg/l (< 2.7 mU/l) during OGTT Age and sex-normalised IGF-I No clinical activity
Inadequately controlled	Nadir GH >1 µg/l (>2.7 mU/l) during OGTT or Elevated IGF-1 Clinically inactive
Poorly controlled	Nadir GH >1 µg/l (>2.7 mU/l) during OGTT Elevated IGF-1 Clinically active

▲ **Figure 5.1** Criteria for cure of acromegaly as formulated by a recent consensus meeting. OGTT, oral glucose tolerance test. (Adapted from Giustina et al. 2000.)

ectopically ACTH-secreting endocrine tumours express SSTR, which in some of these patients allows nonpituitary control of hormonal secretion with SST analogue treatment.

Islet cell tumours and carcinoids also retain characteristics of the cells from which they originate, in that they frequently express SSTRs in most cases. In general, these are slow-growing tumours and the clinical picture of such patients mainly reflects the hypersecretion of hormones. Treatment with SST analogues controls the clinical symptomatology (such as diarrhoea, flushing attacks, hypokalaemia, hypoglycaemic attacks, etc.) in most patients with metastatic hormone-producing carcinoids. In all cases, the number of SSTRs on tumours closely predicts the suppressive effect of chronic therapy with SST analogues on hormonal hypersecretion.

Since SST analogues inhibit the growth of a variety of tumours in different animal models, these compounds have been studied extensively in the treatment of cancer in humans. Despite the direct antimitotic effects of SST analogues on some SSTR-positive breast cancer cell lines, probably because of the nonhomogeneous distribution of SSTRs on most human breast cancer specimens, it has been found that treatment with these compounds affects parts of these tumours only. This implies that a place for SST analogue treatment in patients with SSTR positive breast cancer is not established yet.

The development of somatostatin analogues

The practical use of native SST is hampered by its half-life in the circulation (less than 3 min), and the postinfusion rebound hypersecretion of hormones. As a result of the short half-life of native SST, longer acting and selective SST analogues (octreotide, lanreotide, vapreotide; *Fig. 5.2*) have been developed. These compounds are about 50 times more potent than native SST and have a serum half-life of approximately 2 h after subcutaneous injection.

Somatostatin analogues and receptor subtypes

Octreotide, the first clinically introduced SST analogue, inhibits GH, glucagon and insulin release in monkeys 45, 11 and 1.3 times more actively, respectively, than SS-14. The differential effectiveness of octreotide compared to native SST receptor subtypes must exist to modify hormone secretion in different tissues. The recent cloning of a number of SSTR genes has increased our understanding of its receptor structure and function. To date five human SSTR subtypes have been cloned and characterised. These subtypes belong to a superfamily of receptors that

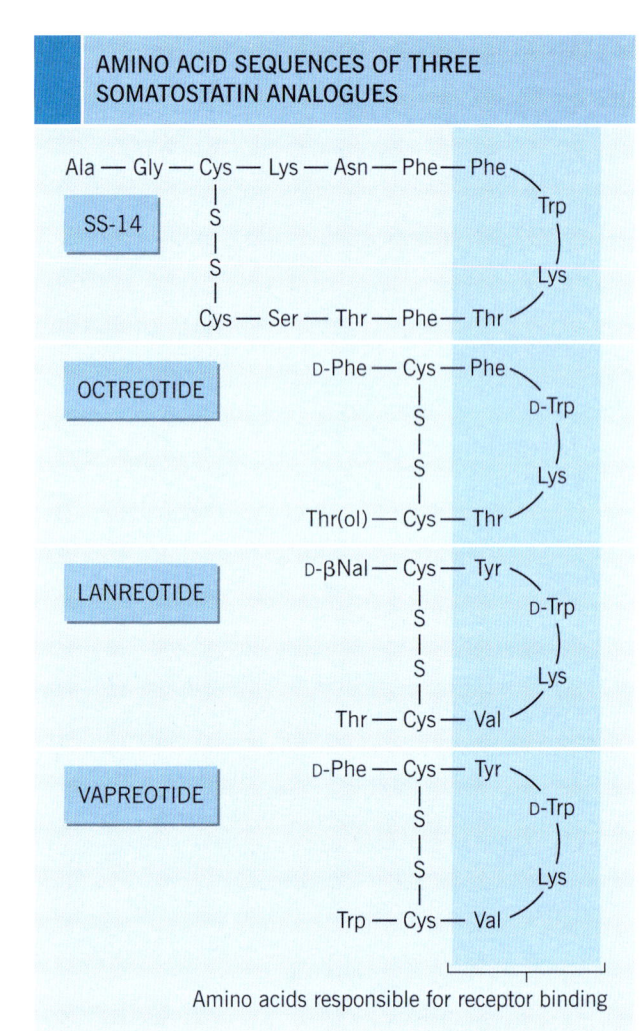

Figure 5.2 Amino acid sequences of the three available somatostatin analogues, compared to endogenous SS-14.

have seven membrane-spanning domains, which are functionally coupled to adenylate cyclase via a pertussis toxin-sensitive G-protein coupled mechanism. Differential coupling between different SSTR subtypes and a variety of intracellular effector systems has been demopnstrated, however. Distinct patterns of expression of these subtypes have been demonstrated, although overlapping expression frequently exists. All five SSTR subtypes bind both SS-14 and SS-28 with a similar high affinity. Octreotide binds with high affinity to SSTR-2, with moderate affinity to SSTR-3 and SSTR-5, and does not bind to SSTR-1 and SSTR-4.

To elucidate the role of the different SSTR subtypes in regulating pituitary hormone secretion, Shimon *et al.* (1997) tested primary human foetal pituitary cells for their responses to SSTR subtype-specific SST analogues, using cultures derived from gestation specimens 23–25 weeks old. They showed that SSTR-2, SSTR-5, GH-releasing hormone and IGF-I receptors are expressed in these foetal cells. Therefore the normal regulators of pituitary GH secretion are already expressed in these cells.

Experimentally promising new SST analogues may be divided into two groups: those that have a high affinity for SSTR-2, as do octreotide and lanreotide (and also BIM-23023, -23190 and -23197), and those that show an increased binding affinity for SSTR-5, as do BIM-23268 and -23052. This new generation of somatostatin analogues offers opportunities to better control hormone hypersecretion in patients with GH-secreting pituitary adenomas, and the future development of novel analogues with improved affinity for both SSTR-2 and SSTR-5 may provide even greater potency to suppress pituitary hormone hypersecretion and perhaps block adenoma growth as well.

Recently, a study using SST analogues preferential for either the SSTR-2 or the SSTR-5 subtype demonstrated a variable suppression of GH and prolactin (PRL) release from GH-secreting adenomas. These data suggested the concept of SSTR-subtype specificity in such tumours. The inhibitory effects of SS-14, octreotide, the SSTR-2 preferential analogue BIM-23197, and the SSTR-5-preferential analogue BIM-23268 on GH and PRL secretion were analysed recently by Jaquet *et al.* (2000) in cells cultured from 15 acromegalic tumours. Although SSTR-5 mRNA was expressed at a higher level than SSTR-2 mRNA, only SSTR-2 mRNA expression correlated with the degree of GH inhibition induced by SS-14, and BIM-23197. The SSTR-5 preferential compound inhibited GH release in only 50% of cases. In cells from mixed adenomas that secreted both GH and PRL, reverse transcriptase (RT) PCR analysis revealed a consistent co-expression of SSTR-5, SSTR-2 and SSTR-1 mRNA. In each case, every analogue with a high affinity for SSTR-5 significantly suppressed PRL secretion. In contrast, the SSTR-2 preferential analogues were effective in suppressing PRL in only 60% of acromegalic tumours. In summary, these data show that SSTR-2 preferential compounds consistently inhibit GH release, whereas SSTR-5 preferential compounds mainly inhibit PRL secretion. When both drugs are combined, they could exert a partial additive inhibitory effect on the co-secretion of both GH and PRL in mixed adenomas, and therefore they may be of interest in the therapeutic approach of this particular type of tumour.

Forms with long-acting application

A form of octreotide with long-acting application has been synthesised; in this 20–30 mg of octreotide is mixed within microspheres of DL-lactide-co-glycolide polymer. This long-acting repeatable (LAR) intramuscular depot preparation of octreotide is well tolerated, and it effectively controls hormonal hypersecretion in most acromegalic patients for 28–42 days. The long-acting intramuscular formulation of lanreotide, which also is bound to lactide–glycolide copolymers in quantities of 30 mg and 60 mg, also effectively controls GH levels in acromegalic patients, but its duration of action is 2 weeks at most. Another long-acting application form of lanreotide, in which lanreotide (60, 90 or 120 mg) is subcutaneously administered in a translucent semisolid form (autogel), will be available in the near future. In clinical studies, this application form effectively controlled GH hypersecretion for at least 4 weeks in acromegalic patients.

Somatostatin analogue therapy of GH-secreting tumours

All the available SST analogues are particularly effective in reducing the headaches often associated with acromegaly. Other features that improve during SST analogue therapy include joint pain, excessive perspiration, cardiomyopathy and sleep apnoea. The subjective clinical benefits of octreotide therapy do not always entirely reflect the decrease in GH and IGF-I levels. A sharp increase in circulating IGF-binding protein-1 (IGFBP-1) levels after octreotide administration has been reported, and it is known that IGFBP-1 inhibits the biological effects of IGF-I on the target cell. We may therefore conclude that an increase in IGFBP-1 levels through SST analogue treatment might have an additional beneficial clinical effect that is not mediated through the pituitary.

Using quality of life (QoL) queries, several studies indicate that treatment with SST analogues significantly improves psychological distress, well-being, and other factors that influence the QoL of patients with acromegaly (e.g. Lamberts *et al.* 1987).

Efficacy of the (long-acting) somatostatin analogues

A number of clinical studies have evaluated the efficacy, tolerability and safety of continuous subcutaneous infusion (CSI) compared to intermittent subcutaneous injection (ISI) of octreotide in the treatment of acromegaly. Normalisation of serum GH or IGF-1 levels, as well as improvement in clinical symptoms, was reported in the majority of the patients for both CSI and ISI. Cases in which pituitary adenomas decreased in size were also documented during the study periods. CSI octreotide gives a better control of GH and IGF-1 than does ISI. CSI octreotide results in similar clinical and biochemical effects at lower doses than ISI octreotide. Finally, the adverse effects with CSI octreotide are reported to be less severe than those with ISI.

The response to clinically available SST analogues is rapid, with GH levels lowered within a few hours. After long-term SSTR ligand administration, GH levels are suppressed to <2.5 µg/l (6.8 mU/l) in 65% of patients. Persistently controlled mean GH levels (<2 µg/l (5.4 mU/l)) are achieved in over 70% of octreotide-sensitive patients. Tumour size is often significantly reduced during long-term treatment with SST analogues, as depicted well in *Figures 5.3* and *5.4*, which clearly show the clinically important tumour shrinkage in two acromegalic patients during long-term subcutaneous octreotide therapy. Slow-release lanreotide (lanreotide-SR) injected every 14 days provides similar GH and IGF-I control. Future treatment options may include receptor-subtype selective SST ligands.

Published efficacy data show a wide range for long-acting application forms of both octreotide and lanreotide. The efficacy of long-acting lanreotide in an Italian multicentre study was reported by Baldelli *et al.* (2000); after 24 months of therapy in 118 patients, control of GH and IGF-I concentration was achieved in 64, 37 and 78% and in 51, 37 and 70% of operated, irradiated, and *de novo* patients, respectively. A reduction in tumour size was documented in 22% of the *de novo* patients. Among the 84 operated and/or irradiated patients with evident tumour remnants, significant shrinkage of these was documented in 6% of patients. Davies *et al.* (1998) evaluated the efficacy and safety of long-acting octreotide in 13 patients with acromegaly for a period of up to 3 years. Long-acting octreotide significantly reduced serum GH and IGF-1 values. For the whole group, mean GH concentrations fell from a baseline of about

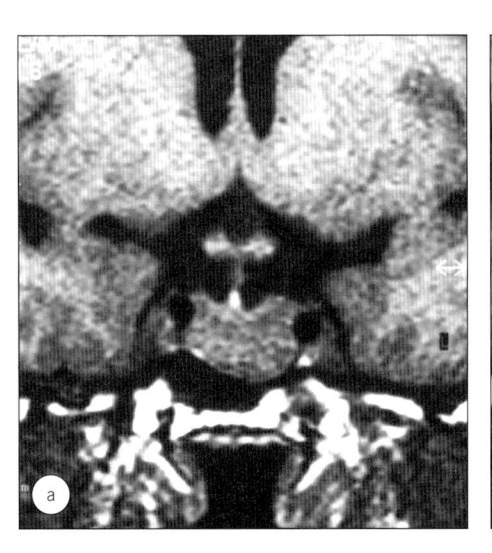

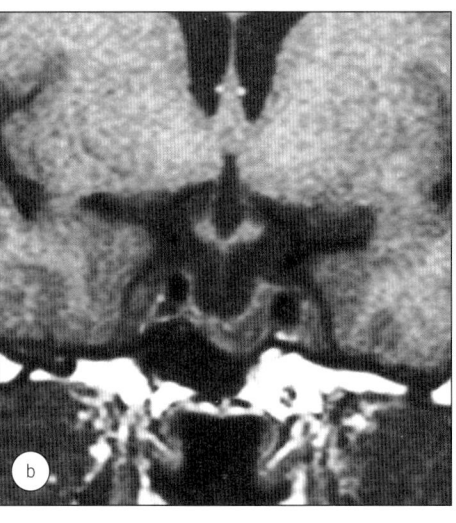

Figure 5.3 (a) A 48-year-old woman with active acromegaly. T1-weighted MRI in the coronal plane showing a pituitary macroadenoma. (b) T1-weighted MRI in the same plane after 3 years of therapy with octreotide 0.1 mg q8h clearly showing tumour shrinkage of the pituitary macroadenoma.

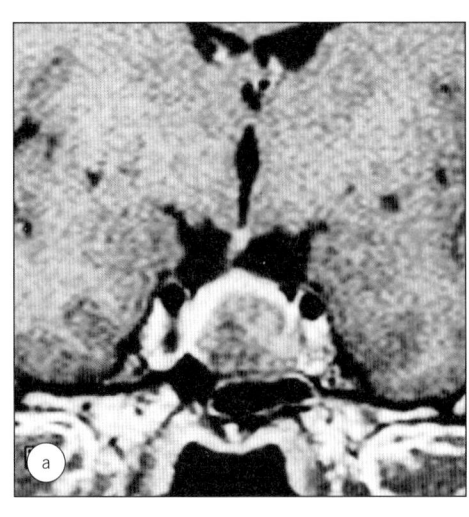

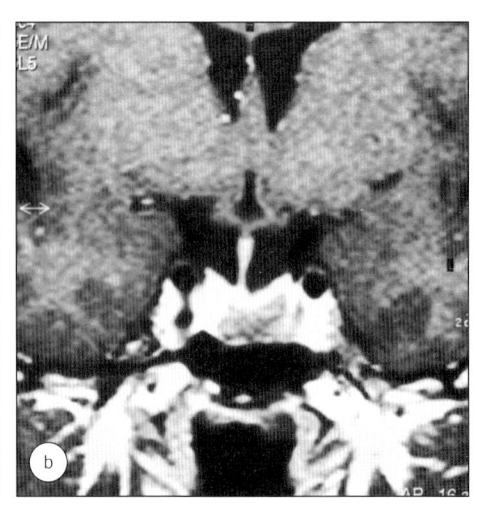

Figure 5.4 (a) A 47-year-old woman with active acromegaly. T1-weighted MRI in the coronal plane after administration of gadolinium-DTPA showing a pituitary macroadenoma. (b) T1-weighted MRI after administration of gadolinium-DTPA after 3 years of therapy with octreotide 0.1 mg q8h clearly showing tumour shrinkage of the pituitary macroadenoma.

9.2 µg/l (25 mU/l) to 1.9 µg/l (5.2 mU/l) at 12 months. In the eight patients treated for 3 years, mean GH levels fell from 10.3 µg/l (28 mU/l) at baseline to 1.5 µg/l (4 mU/l) at the end of 3 years. GH fell to <3.7 µg/l (<10 mU/l) in all subjects and to <1.9 µg/l (<5 mU/l) in 50% after both 1 and 3 years. IGF-1 normalised in 60% of patients after 1 year, and in 75% of patients after 3 years. There was no evidence of tachyphylaxis in any of the available studies on (long-acting) SST analogues.

In a study by Cozzi et al. (1999) of 12 acromegalic patients with active disease sensitive to SST analogues, the efficacies of long-acting release octreotide (octreotide-LAR, administered at 28 day intervals) and lanreotide-SR (administered at 14-day intervals) were compared. After 6–24 months of treatment with lanreotide-SR, patients were switched to treatment with octreotide-LAR, without washout. Both GH and IGF-I concentrations significantly decreased during lanreotide-SR treatment. At the end of the last cycle, octreotide-LAR treatment achieved a significant further suppression in both GH and IGF-I concentrations compared with lanreotide-SR. These data suggest that the once-monthly octreotide-LAR administration schedule is more efficacious than lanreotide-SR given every 7–21 days.

Chanson et al. (2000) compared the efficacy of octreotide-LAR and lanreotide-SR in 125 acromegalic patients. The percentages of patients with mean GH values <2.5 µg/l (<6.8 mU/l) and <1.0 µg/l (<2.7 mU/l) during lanreotide-SR therapy were 54 and 14%, respectively, but these percentages increased after 3 months treatment with octreotide-LAR to 65 and 35% (p <0.001), respectively. The IGF-I levels were normal in 48% of patients at the last evaluation of lanreotide-SR, and in 65% after 3 months on octreotide-LAR (p <0.001). This large multicentre study clearly demonstrates that octreotide-LAR 20 mg administered monthly is more effective in reducing GH and IGF-I in patients with acromegaly than lanreotide-SR administered two or three times monthly. No comparative studies between octreotide-LAR and the newest application form of lanreotide (as an autogel) are available to date (for an overview, see Table 5.1).

Pretreatment of acromegalic patients before neurosurgery

It has been reported that pretreatment with SST analogues in acromegaly improves surgical outcome, although data in the literature are inconsistent. Some studies point out that significant tumour shrinkage occurs during SST analogue treatment in approximately half of the patients, while other studies report tumour shrinkage in a much lower percentage of patients (<20%). Recently, however, an open prospective multicentre trial in the UK (unpublished data) in 27 newly diagnosed untreated acromegalic patients demonstrated that subcutaneous octreotide therapy for 24 weeks (300 µg q8h) induced tumour shrinkage by more than 45%, and a further shrinkage of 37% occurred after the subsequent therapy for 24 weeks

EFFICACY OF LONG-ACTING SOMATOSTATIN ANALOGUES IN ACROMEGALY

Reference	Drug	Efficacy
Morange (1994)	Lanreotide-SR, 30 mg/10–14 days	GH, n: 13/19 (68%) – 0.5 year
Marek et al. (1994)	Lanreotide-SR, 30 mg/14 days	IGF-I, n: 5/10 (50%) – 2 year
Stewart et al. (1995)	Octreotide-LAR, 20–40 mg/month	IGF-I, n: 7/8 (88%) – 1 year
Caron et al. (1995)	Lanreotide-SR, 30 mg/10–14 days	IGF-I, n: 6/9 (66%) – 1 year
Lancranjan et al. (1995)	Octreotide-LAR, 20–40 mg/month	IGF-I, n: 66/101 (65%) – 2 year
Giusti et al. (1996)	Lanreotide-SR, 30 mg/10–14 days	IGF-I, n: 19/50 (38%) – 0.5 year
Flogstad et al. (1997)	Octreotide-LAR, 20–40 mg/month	IGF-I, n: 10/14 (71%) – 1 year
Caron (1997)	Lanreotide-SR, 30 mg/10–14 days	IGF-I, n: 14/22 (63%) – 3 year
Davies et al. (1998)	Octreotide-LAR, 20 mg/month	IGF-I, n: 10/13 (75%) – 3 year
Turner et al. (1999)	Lanreotide-SR, 30 mg/7–10 days	IGF-I, n: 5/9 (56%) – 0.5 year
	Octreotide-LAR, 20 mg/month	IGF-I, n: 7/10 (70%) – 0.5 year
Baldelli et al. (2000)	Lanreotide-SR, 30 mg/10–14 days	IGF-I, n: 24/34 (70%) – 2 year
Chanson et al. (2000)	Lanreotide-SR, 20 mg/10–14 days	IGF-I, n: 53/111 (48%) – 0.25 year
	Octreotide-LAR, 20 mg/month	IGF-I, n: 70/107 (65%) – 0.25 year

Table 5.1 An overview of the available literature on efficacy of the long-acting somatostatin analogues in the treatment of acromegaly.

with long-acting octreotide (20–30 mg monthly). The most important issue is that it is now clear that a short period of treatment with SST analogues improves the clinical condition of acromegalic patients before surgery, especially in terms of cardiac function, blood pressure and glucose and lipid metabolism. Treatment with SST analogues also reduces sleep apnoea. It has been reported that cardiac abnormalities in acromegaly are reversible after suppression of GH hypersecretion. Indeed, a significant decrease in left ventricular mass, interventricular septum thickness and right posterior wall thickness can be found after only 6 months of treatment with (long-acting) SST analogues.

Adverse effects of somatostatin analogue treatment

Initial side effects after the start of SST analogue therapy include abdominal pain, diarrhoea, fat malabsorption, nausea and flatulence. These complaints usually remit spontaneously within 10–14 days, even when treatment continues. This spectrum of adverse effects is readily explained by the physiological actions of SST. The spontaneous resolution of these complaints supports the concept of a rapid adaptation of the functions of the gastrointestinal tract and exocrine pancreas. Bradycardia occurs in approximately 25% of patients, but is considered clinically insignificant. Another side effect associated with SST analogue therapy is an increased risk of asymptomatic cholesterol gallstone development, which occurs in up to 25% of patients. Interestingly, however, the prevalence of octreotide-induced gallstones shows geographical variability, and may be influenced by dietary, environmental or genetic factors. It has been estimated that only approximately 1% of patients per treatment year develop symptoms.

As SST inhibits insulin secretion, a slight deterioration of glucose tolerance is observed in some cases during therapy with octreotide.

In two published case reports diffuse scalp hair loss occurred after several months of therapy with octreotide, which resulted in the discontinuation of treatment (Jonsson and Manhem 1991, Nakauchi *et al*. 1995). After the cessation of octreotide, hair loss stopped and hair growth resumed.

Conclusions

In conclusion, SST analogue therapy induces a fast and effective clinical and biochemical response in the majority of acromegalic patients. Suitable candidates for treatment with these compounds are those patients who have had an unsuccessful transsphenoidal operation, or who await the therapeutic effect of external pituitary irradiation. Elderly acromegalic patients in general demonstrate a higher sensitivity to SST analogues, which suggests that the drug can also be advocated as a primary treatment for this category of patients especially. The decision to treat acromegalic patients with long-acting SST analogues, however, should also be weighed against the adverse effects and costs.

Whether or not the current practice of surgical resection of all newly diagnosed GH-secreting pituitary adenomas, regardless of the likelihood of cure, continues to be advocated remains to be seen. In patients with small (and therefore theoretically resectable) tumours, surgery is probably still the treatment of choice. Also, in patients with relatively high GH concentrations, surgical treatment should be considered as data from the literature indicate that patients with high GH levels are less sensitive to SST analogue treatment when normalisation of IGF-I is used as parameter for efficacy.

DOPAMINE AGONISTS

Introduction

About one-third of the GH-secreting pituitary adenomas are derived from plurihormonal acidophil cells and co-secrete PRL in addition to GH. Dopamine agonists bind to pituitary dopamine type 2 (D2) receptors and suppress GH secretion in some patients with acromegaly. The precise mechanism of action remains unclear. The oldest available dopamine agonist, bromocriptine, provided subjective symptom relief for patients before the availability of any other medical treatments. Tumour shrinkage can be demonstrated in a small minority of patients, although the degree to which these tumours shrink is disappointing.

Bromocriptine

Bromocriptine reduces GH levels, but GH and IGF-I levels are rarely normalised, as less than 20% of patients achieve GH levels <5 µg/l (<13,6 mU/l), and less than 10% of patients achieve normalisation of IGF-I concentrations. An increase in the bromocriptine dose to more than 20 mg/day is not considered to be of clinical advantage.

Quinagolide

The binding of the selective dopamine D2 receptor agonist quinagolide to dopamine D2 receptors is selectively and stereospecifically inhibited by dopamine D2 agents, but not by dopamine D1 compounds. The dopamine D2 receptor selectivity of quinagolide suggested that it might be superior to bromocriptine, especially regarding the side effects mediated by dopamine D1 receptors. The GH inhibitory effect of quinagolide has been studied alone and in combination with octreotide in acromegalic patients. Quinagolide at a dose of 0.3 mg/day normalises GH and IGF-I levels in less than 40% of patients. In roughly 25% of patients the combined therapy of quinagolide and SST analogues induces a greater inhibition of GH and IGF-I levels than does each drug administered alone. Quinagolide is well tolerated by most patients.

Cabergoline

Cabergoline is a long-acting dopamine agonist that is more effective and better tolerated than bromocriptine in patients with acromegaly. Compared to bromocriptine, cabergoline has a more specific D2 receptor-binding capacity and possesses a much longer half-life than bromocriptine. This avoids large fluctuations in dopamine agonist activity, enhances clinical efficacy and reduces side effects, at least in patients with hyperprolactinaemia. As much higher doses of dopamine agonist activity are required for acromegaly than for hyperprolactinaemia, this pharmacological advantage may be of even greater importance. A recent Belgian study by Abs et al. (1998) showed that treatment with cabergoline suppressed plasma IGF-I below 300 μg/l in 39% of cases and between 300 and 450 μg/l in another 28%. An important finding was that in patients with relatively low total serum IGF-I concentrations pretreatment, as well as in those patients with GH and PRL co-secreting adenomas, cabergoline effectively reduced IGF-I levels to the normal range. With pretreatment plasma IGF-I concentrations <750 μg/l, normal IGF-I levels were obtained in 53% of cases. By contrast, with pretreatment plasma IGF-I concentrations >750 μg/l, only 17% of cases showed normalisation of IGF-I levels. For GH and PRL co-secreting adenomas, plasma IGF-I levels were normalised in 50% of cases, but only in about 30% of cases with adenomas that secreted GH only. Except for slight gastrointestinal discomfort and orthostatic hypotension in a few patients at the start of therapy, cabergoline treatment is well tolerated. The weekly dose of cabergoline ranges between 1.0 and 2.0 mg. A further increase in dose is considered not to increase its effectiveness (Table 5.2).

In prolactinoma patients, quinagolide and cabergoline have been compared in terms of effectiveness and tolerability. These studies indicate that with cabergoline the PRL concentrations normalise in a higher percentage of patients during long-term treatment. Clinical response and side effects are similar for both drugs in prolactinoma. In acromegaly, comparative data between quinagolide and cabergoline are scarce.

One study by Colao et al. (1997) reported a comparison of the results of chronic treatment with quinagolide, cabergoline and the no longer available long-acting depot preparation of bromocriptine in 34 acromegalic patients. The chronic administration of these drugs caused a significant decrease of circulating GH, IGF-I and PRL concentrations. Normalisation of circulating GH and IGF-I levels was obtained in 44% of patients treated with quinagolide. Conversely, GH and IGF-I levels did not normalise in any patient treated with either cabergoline or the long-acting depot preparation of bromocriptine therapy. In this study, the percentage of GH suppression during chronic quinagolide and long-acting depot bromocriptine therapy was significantly greater than that obtained during chronic cabergoline treatment (71.4 ± 5.3% and 72.4 ± 3.3% versus 48.5 ± 4.0%). All 34 patients reported a marked improvement of clinical symptoms during treatment with these different dopaminergic agents. Only two patients treated with quinagolide and one with long-acting bromocriptine showed significant tumour shrinkage. Visual field and acuity improved

EFFECT OF CABERGOLINE IN A GROUP OF UNSELECTED ACROMEGALIC PATIENTS

Patients	Baseline IGF–I	Normalisation (%)
Whole group	300–450 μg/l	67
	<300 μg/l	39
Pretreatment IGF-I <750 μg/l	300–450 μg/l	85
	<300 μg/l	53
Pretreatment IGF-I >750 μg/l	300–450 μg/l	38
	<300 μg/l	17
GH and PRL co-secretion	300–450 μg/l	81
	<300 μg/l	50
No PRL co-secretion	300–450 μg/l	62
	<300 μg/l	35

▲ Table 5.2 Cabergoline therapy is more effective in normalising IGF-I levels in patients with relatively low pretreatment serum IGF-I concentrations and in those in whom the somatotropinoma co-secretes both GH and PRL (n = 46, dosages <3.5 mg weekly; mean weekly dose 1–1.5 mg). (Adapted from Abs et al. 1998.)

in all four of the patients who suffered from visual abnormalities. From these data, it was concluded that cabergoline and quinagolide cannot be considered as a useful primary medical approach for most acromegalic patients, as circulating GH and IGF-I levels normalised in only a minority of patients.

Side effects of dopaminergic compounds

Side effects associated with the use of dopaminergic drugs include fatigue, gastrointestinal discomfort (mainly nausea, vomiting and abdominal cramps), nasal stuffiness, arrhythmia, sleep disturbances and postural hypotension. Rarely, peripheral vasospasm is observed.

Sudden somnolence or 'sleep attacks' have been described in parkinsonian patients who take the non-ergoline dopamine agonists. It has been reported that dopaminergic compounds produce psychiatric side effects such as confusion, hallucinations and delusions; a review of the literature supports an anecdotal relationship between psychosis and the use of bromocriptine especially, but also that of quinagolide.

Conclusions

Data from literature suggest that the newer dopaminergic compounds, like quinagolide and cabergoline, can be an effective therapy for acromegaly. The compounds should be considered especially in those patients with a pituitary adenoma that co-secretes GH and PRL and in those patients with pretreatment plasma IGF-I concentrations that do not exceed 750 μg/l.

GROWTH HORMONE ANTAGONISTS

Introduction

The aim of acromegaly treatment is to control the disease by suppressing the clinical and biochemical consequences of GH hypersecretion. Until the late 1990s, nonsurgical treatment options for acromegaly included medical therapy with SST analogues or dopamine agonists and radiotherapy. Thus, until recently the primary goal of treatment for acromegaly was to normalise GH concentrations.

Early studies by Clemmons *et al.* (1980), who utilised high-dose oestrogen therapy, and by Ho *et al.* (1992), who tested the effects of fasting, showed that it is possible to reduce IGF-I concentrations in patients with acromegaly without affecting the concentrations of circulating GH. Although these interventions were clinically impractical, the studies suggested that acromegaly might be treated by disrupting the function of the GH receptor, rather than by attempting to destroy the tumour itself or impairing its secretory capacity.

Before the refinement of GH assays and long-term outcome analyses, GH levels of 2–10 μg/l (5.4–27.2 mU/l) were considered benchmarks of successful therapy. Currently, all patients should experience normal GH levels <1 μg/l (<2.7 mU/l) during treatment with therapies that aim to reduce pathological GH secretion. Approximately 75% of patients with microadenomas and less than 50% of patients with macroadenomas achieve a circulating GH level <2.5 μg/l (< 6.8 mU/l) after surgery. Morbidity and mortality rates remain significantly increased because of a direct deleterious impact of raised GH and IGF-I levels and/or an acromegaly-related co-morbidity, including cardiovascular disease, diabetes, respiratory dysfunction and sleep apnoea. The single most important determinant of mortality in acromegaly seems to be GH levels. Existing epidemiological information strongly suggests that a decrease in GH level in acromegaly is beneficial and may lead to improved or even normal mortality rates. Failure to control GH is associated with a 3.5-fold enhanced mortality. In patients in whom GH is controlled, mortality is no different to that of control groups.

The reported efficacy data of the available long-acting SST analogues in reducing serum IGF-I levels in acromegalic patients indicate that effective control of disease activity can be achieved in two-thirds of patients who are sensitive to SST analogues. Thus, for at least one-third of the patients, medical intervention gives no effective control of disease activity.

Normally, a single molecule of GH binds two GH receptors through sites 1 and 2. When this occurs the receptors dimerise and the GH signal transduction pathway is activated (*Fig. 5.5a*). Pegvisomant, a genetically engineered analogue of GH, increases the binding of the GH receptor to site 1 and blocks the binding at site 2, and so prevents functional GH-receptor dimerisation, initiation of GH action and induction of IGF-I synthesis and secretion (*Fig. 5.5b*). This makes it possible to antagonise the peripheral effects of excess GH at the cellular level, independent of whether SST or dopamine receptors are present on the pituitary tumour. Pegylation of the pegvisomant protein results in a molecule with a long biological half-life of more than 110 h and reduces the likelihood of antibody formation. So pegvisomant is a novel, genetically engineered analogue of hGH that functions as a GH-receptor antagonist. By blocking GH at its site of action, pegvisomant has the potential for greater efficacy

ACTION OF PEGVISOMANT

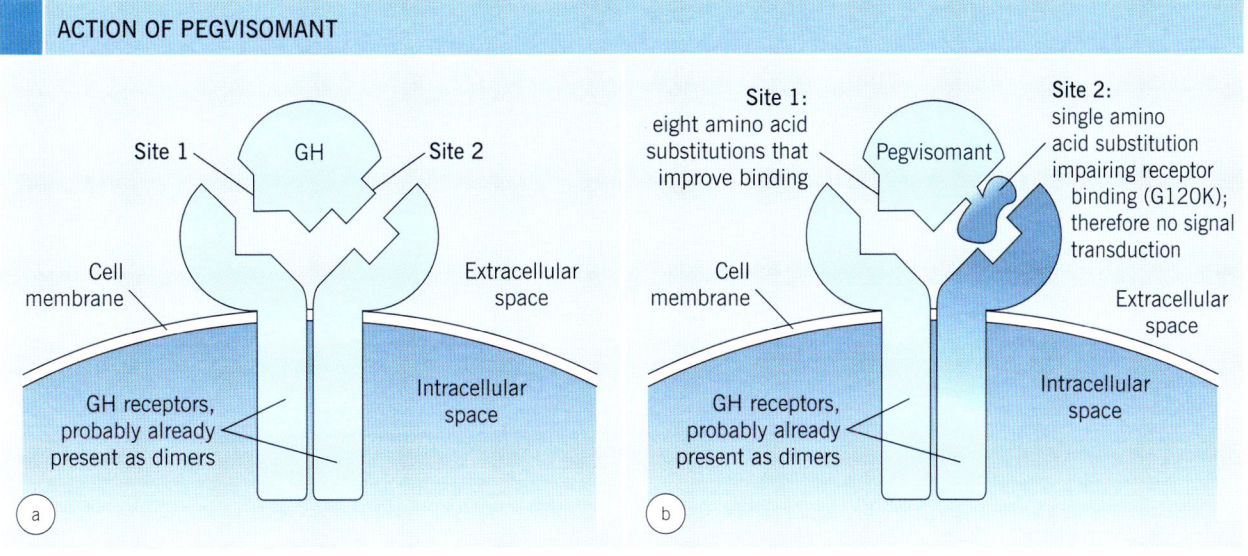

Figure 5.5 (a) Normally a single molecule of GH binds two GH receptors through sites 1 and 2. When this occurs the receptors (probably already present as a dimer) change in configuration and the GH signal transduction pathway is activated. (b) Pegvisomant is engineered to increase binding of GH-receptor to site 1 and block binding at site 2 to prevent functional GH-receptor dimerisation, initiation of GH action and induction of IGF-I synthesis and secretion. This makes it possible to antagonise the peripheral effects of excess GH at the cellular level, independent of the presence of somatostatin or dopamine receptors on the pituitary tumour.

and specificity of action than the current medical treatments for acromegaly. Pegvisomant is a highly selective ligand for the GH receptor, and does not cross-react with other cytokine receptors, including that for PRL. Pegvisomant blocks GH action (i.e. the effect of excess GH at a cellular level), but not GH secretion. On the contrary, it even increases serum GH concentration in a dose-dependent manner. Therefore, the ability to use GH levels as biochemical parameter for the efficacy of treatment is lost.

Efficacy of the GH receptor antagonist

In a 12-week, double-blind, placebo-controlled study, pegvisomant significantly improved both the biochemical and clinical parameters of acromegaly (Trainer et al. 2000). The serum IGF-I of all patients treated with pegvisomant was reduced from baseline in a significant, dose-dependent fashion compared to placebo. Patients treated with the highest dose of pegvisomant in this study (20 mg/day) had a mean reduction in IGF-I of 64%, and 89% of patients achieved a normal IGF-I value at some time during the course of the study and 85% at week 12. The onset of pegvisomant action is rapid and the maximal reduction in IGF-I is achieved within 1 month of therapy initiation. In a report by Herman-Bonert et al. (2000), six patients resistant to maximal doses of octreotide therapy received daily pegvisomant injections of doses determined by titrating IGF-I levels. An important finding was that serum IGF-I concentrations normalised in all six of these acromegalic patients.

Other metabolic consequences of acromegaly may be improved by blocking the GH receptor with pegvisomant. Excess GH, for example, is associated with insulin resistance and patients with acromegaly are insulin resistant. Up to 30% of untreated acromegalic patients have been reported to develop type II diabetes. During long-term treatment with pegvisomant for at least 12 months, fasting serum insulin and glucose concentrations fell significantly. None of these patients, however, were overtly diabetic at baseline. Pegvisomant also influences the development of experimental diabetic nephropathy, which warrants further investigation of the drug's effects on insulin and carbohydrate metabolism in nonacromegalic patients.

Side effects of GH receptor antagonists

Injection site reactions are reported by 10% of patients and are generally mild, erythematous and self-limited reactions that do not require treatment. A local increase in adipose tissue at the injection site has been observed, but only in patients who were administered very high dosages at one site. Two patients showed elevations of alanine aminotransferase and aspartate transaminase more than tenfold the upper normal limit. Both patients showed a normalisation in liver function tests when withdrawn from pegvisomant therapy, with a positive rechallenge in one. No other side effects were reported that could be attributed to the use of pegvisomant. Total serum cholesterol concentrations do not change significantly during the course of pegvisomant treatment. Hypercholesterolaemia is reported as an adverse event in 14% of patients, although most of these patients already had serum total cholesterol concentrations in the upper normal range at baseline.

It has also been postulated that the long-term efficacy of pegvisomant could be compromised by the development of anti-GH or anti-pegvisomant antibodies. Of the more than 150 patients for whom anti-GH antibodies were measured during pegvisomant therapy, 16% had one or more samples test positive. Three patients who experienced sustained low titres of anti-GH antibodies during their course of pegvisomant treatment had normal serum IGF-I concentrations within 2 months of beginning pegvisomant and had normal values for the remainder of their treatment. The presence of pegvisomant in the serum interferes with the assay for anti-pegvisomant antibodies. In 39 patients it was possible, however, to assay for anti-pegvisomant antibodies because these patients were withdrawn from pegvisomant therapy for a period of time. Samples from ten patients tested positive for anti-pegvisomant antibodies (titres ranging from 1:8 to 1:256). In all ten of these patients, anti-GH antibodies were also detected, and the IGF-I levels of nine became normal during pegvisomant treatment, and no tachyphylaxis was observed in any of them.

Serum GH concentrations and the use of GH-receptor antagonists

Serum GH levels increase substantially during pegvisomant therapy. This raises the question whether additional increases in serum GH concentrations might occur during prolonged treatment, as well as whether a sustained increase in serum GH concentrations might overcome the receptor-blocking action of the drug (i.e. induce tachyphylaxis). Also there is the concern that this increase in GH might be accompanied by growth of the pituitary tumour. In principle, an increase in GH concentrations after administration of pegvisomant can be explained by either an increase in GH release and/or production, or a decrease in clearance. Conflicting data on the role of the GH receptor in the process of clearance have been reported. Until pegvisomant became available, it was almost impossible to assess accurately this GH receptor-dependent clearance. Recently, Veldhuis and co-workers (data submitted) addressed this issue. They performed a study in which they showed that pegvisomant fails to impede metabolic removal of endogenous or exogenous GH in healthy adults, using the assessment of endogenous GH half-life by deconvolution analysis in seven adults pretreated with pegvisomant. This finding that the GH receptor apparently does not participate in the *in vivo* GH elimination process is unexpected. It also demonstrates that the observed increase in GH concentrations in both acromegalic patients and normal individuals is likely to result from an increase in release and/or production.

Lamberts *et al.* (1989) demonstrated that both IGF-I and octreotide directly inhibit GH release during a 24 h incubation in, respectively, four and five of seven primary tumour cell cultures, prepared from GH-secreting pituitary adenomas. Interestingly, there seems to be a close correlation between the sensitivity of GH release by cultured human adenoma cells to IGF-I and octreotide. There is also a close correlation between the *in vivo* inhibitory effect on GH release of octreotide and the *in vitro* inhibitory effects of both octreotide and IGF-I. Apparently, many GH-secreting adenomas remain sensitive to the negative feedback effect of IGF-I. The decreased serum IGF-I levels induced by the presence of pegvisomant probably result in a diminished negative feedback of IGF-I on GH release by the pituitary adenoma. This is further supported by the observation that in acromegalic patients who are treated with pegvisomant the rise in mean serum GH concentrations mirrors the fall in serum IGF-I concentrations. Also, GH concentrations increase during the first 2–4 weeks of pegvisomant therapy, but do not continue to increase progressively. In a subgroup of patients (n = 45) who were withdrawn from pegvisomant and not placed on alternative medical therapy for 1 month, the serum GH concentrations decreased to baseline levels, which again strongly suggests that increases in GH concentrations during long-term pegvisomant therapy result from a decrease in the negative feedback effect of high IGF-I levels.

As mentioned above, pegvisomant induces an increase in endogenous serum GH concentrations in both normal individuals and acromegalic patients. The important observation in a patient whose serum IGF-I levels did not normalise while receiving the highest allowed dose of pegvisomant, however, is that lowering serum GH concentrations by octreotide co-administration results in a synergistic decrease in serum IGF-I concentrations that is not achieved with octreotide or pegvisomant alone. This synergistic effect might be predicted because pegvisomant acts as a competitive GH receptor antagonist. Lowering GH levels therefore makes a given concentration of pegvisomant more effective.

Tumour size and the use of GH-receptor antagonists
Paired sets of magnetic resonance imaging (MRI) scans from before and during treatment with pegvisomant are available for more than 130 patients. No statistically significant differences in the change in pituitary tumour volume from baseline could be observed in patients stratified by prior treatment with or without radiation therapy. There was no association between the size of the tumour and the change in tumour volume during pegvisomant therapy. Also, no association was present between the duration of pegvisomant treatment and the change in tumour volume. Two patients, however, demonstrated a clinically significant increase in tumour size while on pegvisomant treatment (neither patient received radiotherapy prior to pegvisomant therapy). One of these patients, the first patient ever treated with pegvisomant, is reported as a case history (van der Lely *et al.* 2001). Furthermore, in this particular patient an increase in tumour size was observed during treatment with pegvisomant. This patient responded to co-treatment of pegvisomant and octreotide, with decreased GH levels, normalisation of serum IGF-I concentrations and improvement of visual field defects.

Conclusions
Pegvisomant is well tolerated. However, that two patients experienced elevations of liver transaminases which required discontinuation of the drug, with a positive rechallenge in one, suggests that caution is warranted and that liver function tests should be regularly monitored until a larger number of patients have been exposed to the drug. The observation that serum IGF-I concentrations fell below the lower limit of the age-adjusted normal range for 11 of the 90 patients treated for more than 1 year, of whom nine required an upward titration of their dose, also suggests that IGF-I must be monitored frequently and the dose adjusted to keep the serum IGF-I concentration within the normal range. Finally, tumour size should be closely followed to detect possible (re)growth of the somatotropinoma during long-term pegvisomant therapy.

THE PLACE OF EACH OF THE MEDICAL TREATMENT MODALITIES

To make a comparison between the most effective treatment modalities for acromegaly, SST analogues and the GH receptor antagonist pegvisomant, several issues should be considered. Such items as control efficacy of biochemical disease activity and clinical disease activity, long-term safety, control of tumour size and mode of administration have to be discussed in this respect (*Table 5.3*).

Efficacy to control biochemical disease activity
It is known that SST analogues effectively normalise serum IGF-I concentrations in about two-thirds of acromegalic patients, although the reported

COMPARISON OF ACROMEGALY TREATMENT MODALITIES

SST analogues	Pegvisomant
Effective in about 65% of cases	Effective in about 100% of cases
Considered to reduce clinical symptomatology	Proved to reduce clinical symptomatology
Long-term safety known	Long-term safety unknown
Effective tumour-size control	Long-term effect on tumour size unknown
(Bi)monthly injections (s.c. or i.m.)	Daily s.c. injections

▲ Table 5.3 A comparison between the most effective treatment modalities for acromegaly, SST analogues and the GH receptor antagonist pegvisomant, on control efficacy of biochemical disease activity, clinical disease activity, long-term safety, control of tumour size and mode of administration.

effectiveness in reducing IGF-I levels ranges from 50 to 75%. Pegvisomant, however, is able to reduce serum IGF-I concentrations in virtually all acromegalic patients. This is certainly true if the dose of pegvisomant is increased, as expected for a competitive receptor blocker that competes with the endogenous ligand. In this respect, pegvisomant is superior to any available treatment modality for acromegaly, both surgical or medical. However, pegvisomant induces an increase in endogenous GH concentrations while blocking the GH action. This implies that GH concentrations cannot be used as a parameter to assess, for example, the long-term sequelae of acromegaly. No studies that use IGF-I as a parameter of morbidity and mortality data in acromegaly are available yet. Therefore, it will be difficult to compare the long-term safety data on pegvisomant therapy with that of other treatment modalities, including surgery and radiotherapy.

Another issue is that we do not know whether future developments in SST analogues that have a higher affinity for both SSTR-2 and SSTR-5 receptors will increase the efficacy with which SST analogues normalise serum IGF-I concentrations.

Efficacy to control clinical disease activity

Strange as it may be, and despite the amount of safety data and the well-known clinical experience of many clinicians, only a few actual data exist on the improvement in clinical disease activity of acromegalic patients while being treated with SST analogues. However, pegvisomant treatment induces a clear-cut improvement in clinical signs and symptoms. These improvements can readily be demonstrated within 3 months of therapy and they are also dose dependent.

Long-term safety

Obviously, many more data are available concerning the safety of current SST analogues than that of pegvisomant in the long-term treatment of acromegaly. It is clear that SST analogues can be considered very safe, and induce clinical signs and symptoms of gallstone formation in only a handful of patients. Safety data on the adverse effects of pegvisomant are scarce. Clinical experience with pegvisomant, however, extends now to an accumulated 186 patient-years of exposure, with each patient being treated for an average of more than 400 days. One potential concern with regard to safety is the observation of clinically important liver function abnormalities in two patients. Therefore, it is advocated that liver functions be checked on a regular basis during long-term treatment with pegvisomant.

Effective tumour size control

In general, the size of GH-producing pituitary tumours decreases during therapy with SST analogues. However, patients for whom SST analogues do not effectively control the signs and symptoms of acromegaly are subsequently operated upon, as are those in whom serum GH and IGF-I concentrations remain elevated despite high doses of SST analogues. After neurosurgery, radiotherapy is frequently applied to prevent regrowth of the tumour remnant. Long-term data on changes in tumour size during pegvisomant therapy are available from paired sets of MRIs in about 130 patients. In these patients, the mean duration of pegvisomant treatment at the time of the most recent scan for this group was 1 year, ranging from a minimum of 6 weeks to a maximum of 2.5 years. There was no association between size of the tumour and change in tumour volume while on pegvisomant therapy, nor was there an association between the duration of pegvisomant treatment and change in tumour volume. In this relatively short period of treatment, as far as tumour (re)growth is concerned only two patients required treatment because of a clinically important progression in tumour size. Both already had large, globular tumours at baseline, with impingement on the optic chiasm. Whether pegvisomant treatment does not interfere with the natural history of these GH-producing tumours or, in fact, induces an increase in the size of a tumour by increasing GH secretion remains unclear.

Differences in administration method

As a consequence of the nature of these compounds, both SST analogues and pegvisomant have to be administered either subcutaneously or intramuscularly. Pegvisomant needs daily injections, although its half-life of more than 120 h should allow a longer interval between injections. However, through concentrations are higher when pegvisomant is given daily instead of weekly, and so the efficacy of daily injections has proved superior to that of weekly administrations. Both octreotide-LAR and lanreotide-SR must be administered intramuscularly at intervals of 7–14 days (lanreotide-SR) or 4 weeks (octreotide-LAR). When lanreotide autogel becomes available, it can be given once monthly. The advantage of lanreotide autogel is that it can be given subcutaneously and so can be self-administered.

How to treat acromegalic patients with medication

The approach to treatment is summarised in *Box 5.1* and also in *Figure 5.6*.

Box 5.1 Approaches to treatment

- Taking into account all the factors discussed, SST analogues are currently considered the first choice of treatment for acromegalic patients for whom medical treatment is indicated. Although the available SST analogues are less effective than pegvisomant in normalising total serum IGF-I concentrations, their safety record makes them the first-line medical treatment.
- Only in acromegalic patients for whom serum IGF-I levels are relatively low, or in whom GH and PRL co-secretion is present, should dopaminergic compounds, such as quinagolide and cabergoline, be used to control biochemical and clinical disease activity.
- When treatment with SST analogues has commenced, but patients show no clinically significant reduction in serum IGF-I concentrations, pegvisomant should be started. In such cases, tumour size should be closely followed, as well as liver function. Whether or not follow up of the measurement of GH concentrations is necessary is not clear; the available data suggest that increases in GH during pegvisomant treatment are likely to occur within 1 month, and thereafter they remain stable in general. The clinical significance of these increases in serum GH concentrations, however, is far from clear, as they do not correlate with any other parameter, tumour size included. With this doubt, it seems advisable to continue SST analogue administration together with low-dose pegvisomant.
- If the side effects of the long-term use of SST analogues are still present after 6 months and to such an extent that both the patient and the physician consider discontinuation of SST analogue therapy appropriate, pegvisomant treatment should be commenced. The safety parameters described herein apply.

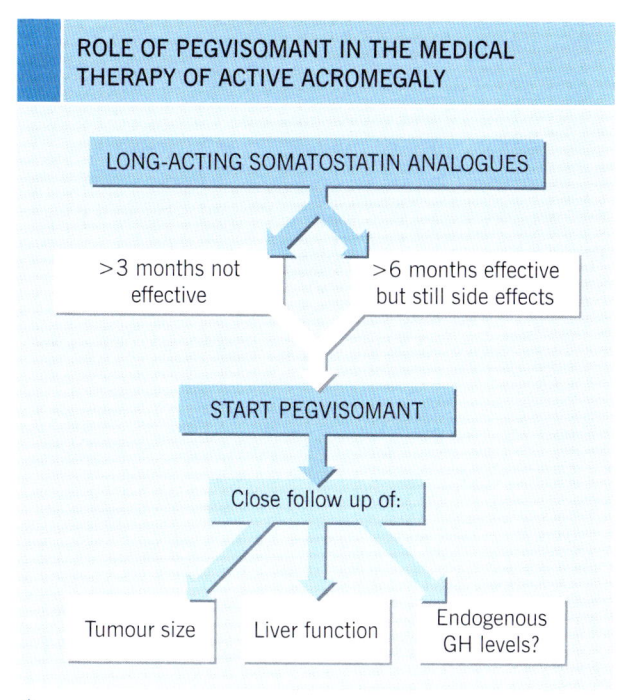

Figure 5.6 The role of pegvisomant in the medical therapy of active acromegaly.

References

Abs R, Verhelst J, Maiter D et al. 1998 Cabergoline in the treatment of acromegaly: a study in 64 patients. *Journal of Clinical Endocrinology and Metabolism* **83** 374–378.

Baldelli R, Colao A, Razzore P et al. 2000 Two-year follow-up of acromegalic patients treated with slow release lanreotide (30 mg). *Journal of Clinical Endocrinology and Metabolism* **85** 4099–4103.

Caron P, Cogne M, Gusthiot-Joudet B, Wakim S, Catus F & Bayard F 1995 Intramuscular injections of slow-release lanreotide (BIM 23014) in acromegalic patients previously treated with continuous subcutaneous infusion of octreotide (SMS 201-995) *European Journal of Endocrinology* **132** 320–325.

Caron P, Morange-Ramos I, Cogne M & Jaquet P 1997 Three year follow-up of acromegalic patients treated with intramuscular slow-release lanreotide. *Journal of Clinincal Endocrinology and Metabolism* **82** 18–22.

Chanson P, Boerlin V, Ajzenberg C et al. 2000 Comparison of octreotide acetate LAR and lanreotide SR in patients with acromegaly. *Clinical Endocrinology (Oxford)* **53** 577–586.

Clemmons DR, Underwood LE, Ridgway EC et al. 1980 Estradiol treatment of acromegaly. Reduction of immunoreactive somatomedin-C and improvement in metabolic status. *American Journal of Medicine* **69** 571–575.

Colao A, Ferone D, Marzullo P et al. 1997 Effect of different dopaminergic agents in the treatment of acromegaly. *Journal of Clinical Endocrinology and Metabolism* **82** 518–523.

Cozzi R, Dallabonzana D, Attanasio R, Barausse M & Oppizzi G 1999 A comparison between octreotide-LAR and lanreotide-SR in the chronic treatment of acromegaly. *European Journal of Endocrinology* **141** 267–271.

Davies PH, Stewart SE, Lancranjan L, Sheppard MC & Stewart PM 1998 Long-term therapy with long-acting octreotide (Sandostatin-LAR) for the management of acromegaly. *Clinical Endocrinology (Oxford)* **48** 311–316.

Flogstad AK, Halse J, Bakke S et al. 1997 Sandostatin LAR in acromegalic patients: long-term treatment. *Journal of Clinical Endocrinology and Metabolism* **82** 23–28.

Giusti M, Gussoni G, Cuttica CM, Giordano G, & the Italian Multicentre Slow Release Lanreotide Study Group 1996 Effectiveness and tolerability of slow release lanreotide treatment in active acromegaly: six-month report on an Italian multicenter study. *Journal of Clinical Endocrinology and Metabolism* **81** 2089–2124.

Giustina A, Barkan A, Casanueva FF *et al*. 2000 Criteria for cure of acromegaly: a consensus statement. *Journal of Clinical Endocrinology and Metabolism* **85** 526–529.

Herman-Bonert VS, Zib K, Scarlett JA & Melmed S 2000 Growth hormone receptor antagonist therapy in acromegalic patients resistant to somatostatin analogs. *Journal of Clinical Endocrinology and Metabolism* **85** 2958–2961.

Ho PJ, Friberg RD & Barkan AL 1992 Regulation of pulsatile growth hormone secretion by fasting in normal subjects and patients with acromegaly. *Journal of Clinical Endocrinology and Metabolism* **75** 812–819.

Jaquet P, Saveanu A, Gunz G *et al*. 2000 Human somatostatin receptor subtypes in acromegaly: distinct patterns of messenger ribonucleic acid expression and hormone suppression identify different tumoral phenotypes. *Journal of Clinical Endocrinology and Metabolism* **85** 781–792.

Jonsson A & Manhem P 1991 Octreotide and loss of scalp hair. *Annals of Internal Medicine* **115** 913.

Lamberts SW, Uitterlinden P, & Del Pozo E 1987 SMS 201-995 induces a continuous decline in circulating growth hormone and somatomedin-C levels during therapy of acromegalic patients for over two years. *Journal of Clinical Endocrinology and Metabolism* **65** 703–710.

Lamberts SW, van Koetsveld P & Hofland L 1989 A close correlation between the inhibitory effects of insulin-like growth factor-I and SMS 201-995 on growth hormone release by acromegalic pituitary tumours *in vitro* and *in vivo*. *Clinical Endocrinology (Oxford)* **31** 401–410.

Lamberts SW, van der Lely AJ, de Herder WW & Hofland LJ 1996 Octreotide. *New England Journal of Medicine* **334** 246–254.

Lancranjan I, Bruns C, Grass P *et al*. 1996 Sandostatin LAR: a promising therapeutic tool in the management of acromegalic patients. *Metabolism* **45** (Suppl 1) 67–71.

Marek J, Hana V, Krsek M, Justova V, Catus F & Thomas F 1994 Long-term treatment of acromegaly with the slow-release somatostatin analogue lanreotide. *European Journal of Endocrinology* **131** 20–26.

Melmed S, Jackson I, Kleinberg D & Klibanski A 1998 Current treatment guidelines for acromegaly. *Journal of Clinical Endocrinology and Metabolism* **83** 2646–2652.

Morange I, De Boisvilliers F, Chanson P *et al*. 1994 Slow release lanreotide treatment in acromegalic patients previously normalized by octreotide. *Journal of Clinical Endocrinology and Metabolism* **79** 145–151.

Nakauchi Y, Kumon Y, Yamasaki H, Tahara K, Kurisaka M & Hashimoto K 1995 Scalp hair loss caused by octreotide in a patient with acromegaly: a case report. *Endocrinology Journal* **42** 385–389.

Shimon JE, Taylor JZ, Dong RA *et al*. 1997 Somatostatin receptor subtype specificity in human fetal pituitary cultures. Differential role of SSTR-2 and SSTR-5 for growth hormone, thyroid-stimulating hormone, and prolactin regulation. *Journal of Clinical Investigation* **99** 789–798.

Stewart PM, Kane KF, Stewart SE, Lancranjan I & Sheppard MC 1995 Depot long-acting somatostatin analog (Sandostatin-LAR) is an effective treatment for acromegaly. *Journal of Clinical Endocrinology and Metabolism* **80** 3267–3272.

Trainer PJ, Drake WM, Katznelson L *et al*. 2000 Treatment of acromegaly with the growth hormone-receptor antagonist pegvisomant. *New England Journal of Medicine* **342** 1171–1177.

Turner HE, Vadivale A, Keenan J & Wass JAH 1999 A comparison of lanreotide and octreotide LAR for treatment of acromegaly. *Clinical Endocrinology (Oxford)* **51** 275–280.

van der Lely AJ, Muller AF, Janssen JA 2001 Control of tumor size and disease activity during co-treatment with octreotide and the growth hormone receptor antagonist pegvisomant in an acromegalic patient. *Journal of Clinical Endocrinology and Metabolism* **86** 478–481.

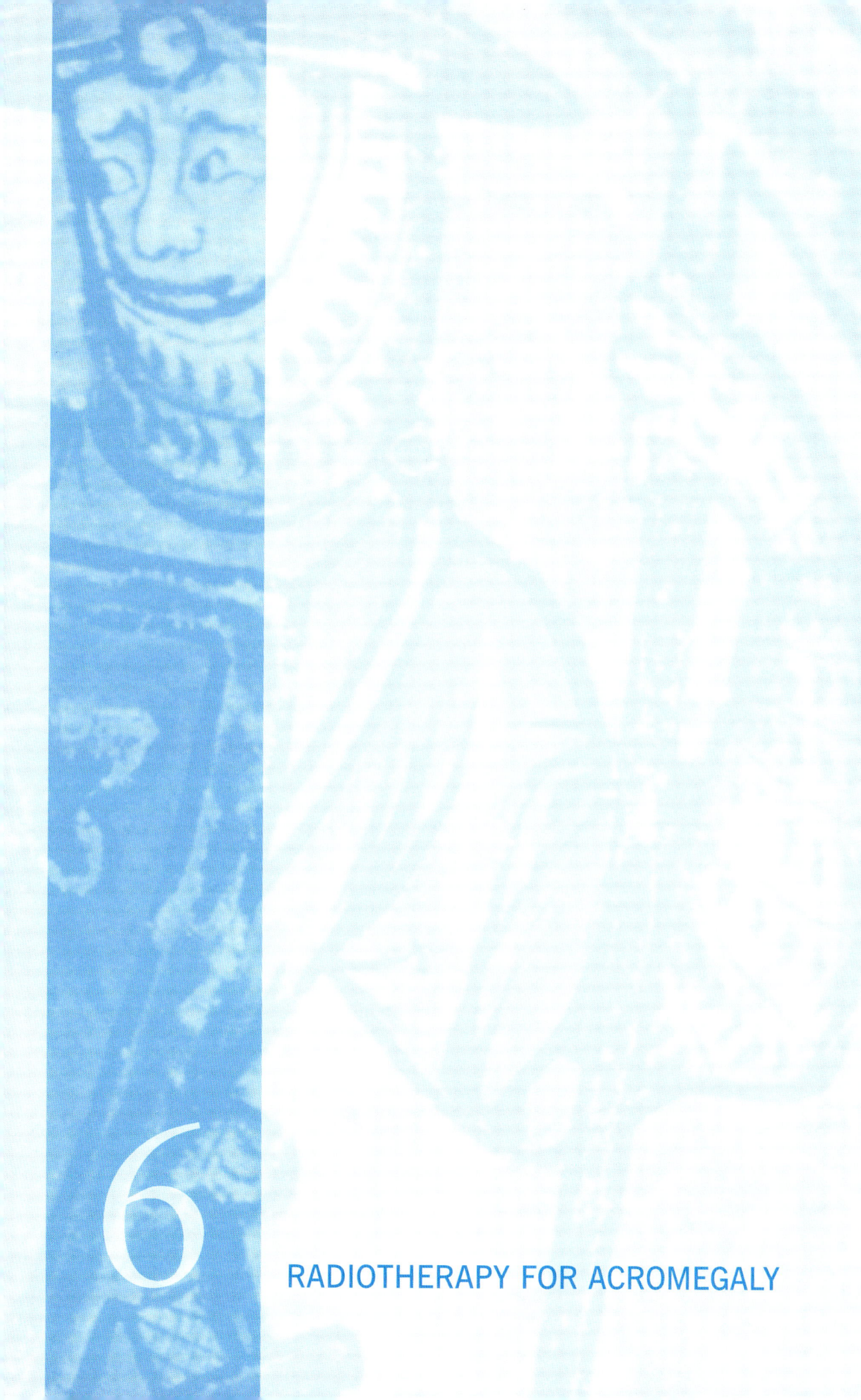

6

RADIOTHERAPY FOR ACROMEGALY

6 RADIOTHERAPY FOR ACROMEGALY

Paul J Jenkins Department of Endocrinology, St Bartholomew's and The Royal London Hospital, London, UK

P Nicholas Plowman Department of Radiotherapy, St Bartholomew's and The Royal London Hospital, London, UK

INTRODUCTION

Radiotherapy has a long track record in the effective therapy of pituitary adenoma. In 1909 Béclère published his now famous case report entitled *The radiotherapeutic treatment of tumours of the hypophysis, gigantism and acromegaly*. In this paper he describes his first case:

A young girl of sixteen suffering from hypophysomegaly. The X-rays showed a notable enlargement of the sella turcica. She suffers from violent attacks of cephalalgia, severe visual troubles, gigantism, genital infantilism and excess adiposity ...

and concerning radiotherapy:

The séances have now been carried out once a week for ten weeks. At each séance, the hypophysis was treated by cross fire through four or five different areas on the fronto-temporal region, the skin dose on each being 3H. The attacks of cephalalgia have completely disappeared. Still important is the improvement in the visual troubles.

Subsequent to this seminal report, a number of different modalities to administer pituitary radiotherapy were developed, although it was not until the 1970s that pituitary irradiation became standard therapy in acromegaly. With increasing experience and critical analysis most of these modalities, such as yttrium implants and charged particle beams (protons), are no longer in routine use and for the past 30 years almost every centre has used megavoltage X-ray therapy.

THEORETICAL ASPECTS

The term radiotherapy refers to the delivery of ionising radiation onto tumours to arrest their growth by sterilising their component cells, but not destroying the structure or function of the surrounding normal tissues. As cellular damage mediated by ionising radiation is not tumour selective, the thrust of successful modern radiotherapy has been towards improving the therapeutic ratio and clinical effectiveness.

The first and most obvious objective is to deposit more radiation on the tumour than on the normal surrounding structures – this improvement in clinical effectiveness is achieved by careful radiotherapy planning. In the treatment of pituitary adenoma, it is usual practice to make an individually constructed plastic mask to immobilise the patient's head and then bring in at least three beams from different directions to cross-fire the pituitary and so concentrate the dose on this target, while reducing the dose to the surrounding structures, which do not lie in the cross-fire region. We employ modern linear accelerators that generate deeply penetrating megavoltage X-ray beams. These beams result in higher depth doses per unit surface dose as compared to the old-fashioned orthovoltage/deep X-ray treatment (DXT). The modern megavoltage X-ray beams are also much better collimated (less side scatter) than DXT radiation beams. The three administered fields comprise an antero-oblique and two lateral portals, which cross-fire on the individually mapped (magnetic resonance imaging (MRI)) tumour. By this methodology, a high dose is deposited on the target, whereas the adjacent brain (e.g. temporal lobes) receives a much lower dose (*Fig. 6.1*). Focal methods of radiation therapy other than the so-called conventional radiotherapy just described are known as radiosurgical methods, because of the concept that the stereotactic mapping and precise ablative deposition of the radiation dose is akin to the surgical knife ablation of targets (see below and *Fig. 6.1*).

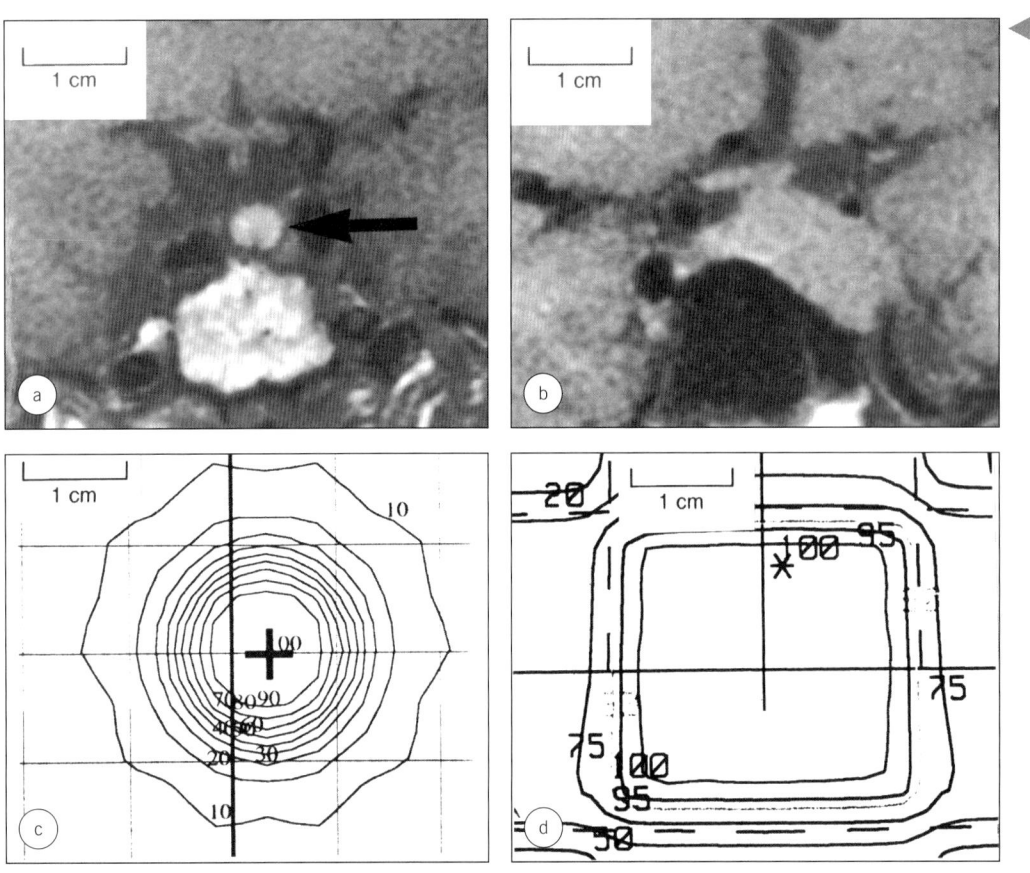

Figure 6.1
(a, b) Coronal MRI of two patients with pituitary adenoma. (a) The patient has a small, discrete, low lying adenoma, whereas the patient in (b) has a large tumour extending into the adjacent cavernous sinus. (c) Radiosurgical isodosimetry used to treat the small adenoma (a). (d) Broader coverage of conventional, three-field planning radiotherapy. Note the faster 'fall off' of dose at the margins of the radiosurgical target volume.

The second feature to improve the clinical effectiveness of radiotherapy is delivery of the total radiation dose in a large number of small daily doses – 'fractionation'. It has been known for some 80 years that fractionation of a dose of radiotherapy allows more 'normal tissue sparing' than tumour sparing (because normal tissues are under homeostatic influences that sense and respond to cellular damage/depletion; tumours have lost these homeostatic recovery processes). When pituitary radiotherapy is recommended (under current guidelines for acromegaly this includes those patients with a mean serum growth hormone (GH) level >5 mU/l (>2.5 μg/l)), it is our policy to select conventionally fractionated radiotherapy. In this radiotherapy the beam is concentrated on the target volume (the whole fossa and any tumour extension beyond) by the 'cross-fire' technique just described and with the patient immobilised in a tight-fitting mask. The portals may be manipulated to conform to irregular-shaped volumes. Over the years, we have established an optimal dose prescription for the radiotherapy of pituitary adenoma, which comprises a total dose of 45 Gy in 25 fractions of 1.8 Gy given every week day (i.e. 5 days a week) for 5 weeks. This dose prescription is highly effective at controlling the growth of pituitary adenoma and the secretion of GH and yet is 'kind' to the optic chiasm and other adjacent sensitive structures.

In 'radiosurgery', the extreme focal nature of the deposition of the radiation dose may allow the clinician to deposit a large single dose of radiation on the target, without worrying about the need to fractionate, because the dose 'fall-off' at the edge of the target is so fast that only a small percentage of the dose is received by the surrounding structures (see below and *Fig. 6.1*).

EFFECTS ON GROWTH HORMONE AND INSULIN-LIKE GROWTH FACTOR-I

Since the initial description by Béclère, numerous studies have confirmed the efficacy of external pituitary irradiation as a treatment for acromegaly. However, early reports relied upon a subjective improvement in symptoms as a measure of success and it was not until the development of a radioimmunoassay for GH that objective benefits of irradiation could be documented.

In 1981, Sheline described a 25% recurrence-free survival rate at 5 years and 9% at 10 years following transcranial surgery performed for pituitary adenoma in the era prior to modern computed tomography (CT) or MRI; however, with postoperative radiotherapy, the recurrence-free survival at 10 years was 79%. In the more modern era, Brada et al. (1993) found an actuarial progression-free survival rate of 94% at 5 and 88% at 10 years (slightly worse control rates for secretory than nonfunctioning adenomas) with the routine use of postoperative radiotherapy.

At St Bartholomew's Hospital, the conventional external-beam radiotherapy technique and prescription has been in routine use for more than 30 years and our results in acromegaly have been published and are typical of the findings of others. Ciccarelli et al. (1988) carefully followed 73 patients with acromegaly (61 unoperated and 12 postoperative cases) who had been treated by our three-field linear accelerator technique to a dose of 45 Gy in 25 fractions over 35 days – all GH data points were made when off medical therapy. The importance of this series, now over a decade from first reporting, is that some relatively advanced cases were included. Thus, the mean serum GH level was 103 ± 14 mU/l (51.5 ± 7 µg/l) prior to radiotherapy. Following radiotherapy, a slow but progressive decline in the GH level occurred over the next decade such that the mean GH level at the 10-year follow-up point was 12.2 ± 2.4 mU/l (6.1 ± 1.2 µg/l). Furthermore, in 31 patients who had been followed for more than 10 years, there was a significant further fall in GH in the next 5 years.

Although this and other studies all demonstrate that pituitary radiotherapy results in a reduction in serum GH levels, there are differences between series in the efficacy and proportion of patients who achieve a 'cure'. Such differences arise from a number of factors.

- The most important variables between series relate to differences in the mean baseline pre-irradiation GH level and to variations in duration of follow up.
- The majority of series involved small numbers of patients, especially with regard to long-term results.
- A lack of uniformity not only in the modality by which irradiation was administered and the total dose, but also in the radioimmunoassays used to measure both GH and, more recently, serum insulin-like growth factor-I (IGF-I).
- Differences in the rate of long-term ascertainment. A low rate of follow up may reflect a selection bias towards those patients with poor outcome and thus ongoing symptoms, which are likely to reflect high biochemical activity.

- Early studies utilised suboptimal imaging techniques, which would have resulted in imprecise dosimetry. Modern MRI or CT enables accurate delineation of the adenoma margins and thus more focused dosimetry.
- A variety of different criteria for 'cure' have been used. The majority of early studies used a target GH level <10 mU/l (<5 µg/l) as representing a satisfactory outcome, whereas it is now generally accepted that a level <5mU/l (<2.5 µg/l) should be the aim, as such a level is associated with a reduction in morbidity and restoration of mortality rates towards those of the nonacromegalic population.

Notwithstanding these differences, most studies consistently demonstrate that within the first 2 years after pituitary irradiation there is approximately a 50% decline in baseline serum GH levels, and a 75% decrease at 5 years. Long-term follow up of patients has revealed that this decline continues in an exponential manner for more than 20 years.

These figures are exemplified by data from the largest study, to date, of the effects of pituitary irradiation in acromegaly (Jenkins et al. 1999). Data were collected from several centres in the UK (UK National Acromegaly Study Group) for a total of 372 patients who had received pituitary irradiation. The mean baseline GH level was 24.2 mU/l (12.1 µg/l), which declined to 12.5 mU/l (6.25 µg/l) at 2 years and 7.8 mU/l (3.9 µg/l) at 5 years. Among all patients, a target level <5 mU/l (<2.5 µg/l) was achieved in 36% of patients at 2 years, 44% at 5 years, 59% at 10 years and 100% after 20 years follow up (*Fig. 6.2*).

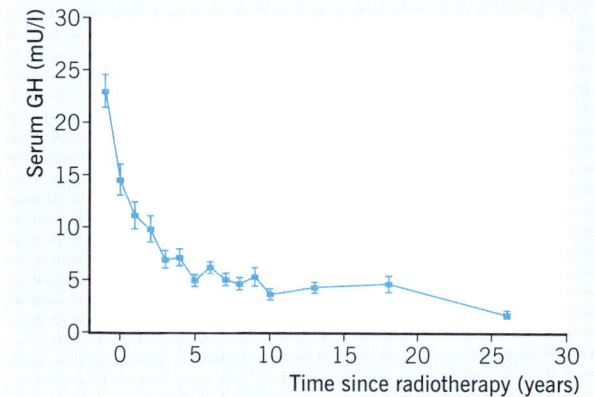

Figure 6.2 Effects of conventional radiotherapy on mean serum GH levels of a large cohort of acromegalic patients. Data from the UK National Acromegaly Study Group.

Several factors affect the eventual success of pituitary irradiation:
- Given that at least a 50% decline occurs in GH levels within the first 2 years, the predominant determinant to the eventual success is the initial baseline serum GH level. In the UK series, of the patients with an initial serum GH <10 mU/l (<5 μg/l), 70% achieved a level <5 mU/l (<2.5 μg/l) after a mean interval of 1.7 years; 45% of those with an initial level between 10 and 30 mU/l (5 and 15 μg/l) achieved this level after a mean of 4.7 years, while 31% of those who had an initial level >60 mU/l (>30 μg/l) achieved a safe level after a mean of 7.6 years (Fig. 6.3).
- The size of the pituitary tumour. Not only is there a correlation between GH levels and adenoma size, but a large invasive macroadenoma is more difficult to encompass within irradiation fields than an intrasellar microadenoma.
- Prior pituitary surgery can minimise each of these factors by reducing both the tumour mass and baseline GH levels, and thus improve irradiation outcome.
- The dose of irradiation is also important. An early study by Sheline (1981) demonstrated that a total dose <40 Gy was less effective than a dose ≥ 40 Gy. Although, in contrast, Littley et al. (1990) later reported that a total dose of 20 Gy was as effective as the conventional dose in reducing serum GH levels, they did not take into account the radiobiological dose, which is a combination of both total dose and daily fraction dose. Their daily fraction was 2.5 Gy, which is significantly higher than the 1.8–2.0 Gy currently recommended by most centres. In terms of reducing risks to the adjacent nervous system, most workers would nowadays prefer to use the lower daily dose fractions.

There appears to be no difference between pure GH-secreting tumours and those that secrete both GH and prolactin (PRL) in the GH response to radiation. However, the responses of PRL itself to irradiation are variable. Ciccarelli et al. (1989) demonstrated that the majority of patients with normal PRL levels at baseline show a significant rise in serum PRL after irradiation, with the peak occurring at 1–6 years, after which levels progressively decline to normal. However, in contrast, approximately 40% of patients with an elevated baseline PRL level demonstrate the opposite, with serum levels falling in response to irradiation.

Effects on IGF-I measurements

Following the introduction of a radioimmunoassay for IGF-I, some authors advocated that measurement of circulating IGF-I levels should be substituted for that of GH in the assessment of GH secretion in acromegaly. However, although convenient – being a single measurement – such an approach is not without its limitations. While there is a statistical correlation between a single IGF-I level and the mean value of several GH measurements taken over a period of 10–12 h (a so-called day curve, which is the generally accepted 'gold standard' method of assessment), it should be remembered that many other factors also affect hepatic IGF-I secretion, including sex, age and nutrition. Several series have reported discordance between serum GH and IGF-I levels, either with a 'normal' mean GH level and elevated IGF-I or vice versa. Furthermore, recent evidence strongly suggests that paracrine–autocrine IGF-I rather than hepatic-derived peptide is responsible for most of the growth-promoting effects of GH. Therefore, serum IGF-I levels should be used more as a marker of pituitary GH secretion than as a substitute.

Notwithstanding these points, the effects of pituitary irradiation on reducing circulating IGF-I levels have been unclear. In a recent series, normalisation of IGF-I levels was achieved in a disappointing 5% of irradiated patients. However, several factors may have accounted for this poor result:
- low numbers of patients studied;
- lack of uniformity in the IGF-I assays and irradiation techniques; and
- short duration of follow up.

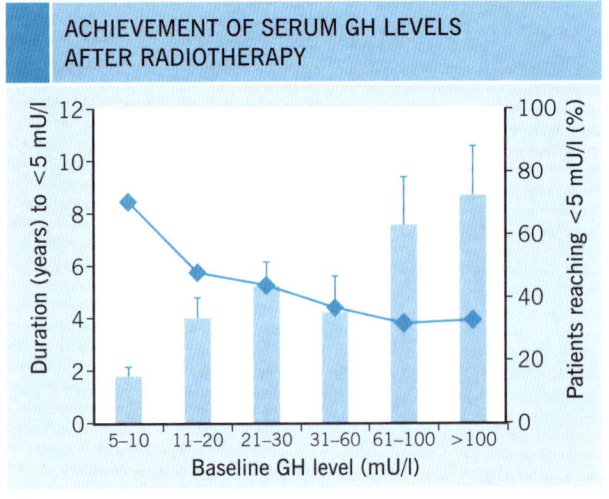

Figure 6.3 The proportion of acromegalic patients (curve) and the mean interval (bar chart) to achieve a serum GH level <5 mU/l (<2.5 μg/l) after radiotherapy according to baseline GH levels.

Several subsequent studies confirmed the efficacy of pituitary irradiation in reducing circulating IGF-I levels. Powell *et al.* (2000) reported that more than 60% of patients achieved a normal IGF-I level at 10 years, which increased to 80% of patients after further long-term follow up. These results were confirmed in another recent study, which recorded a normal IGF-I level in 70% of patients at 10 years and 84% at 15 years (Biermasz *et al.* 2000). Data from the UK National Acromegaly Study Group also support a beneficial effect of irradiation in reducing serum IGF-I levels in parallel with those of GH, with normalisation of serum IGF-I occurring in 27% of patients after 3 years, 53% after 7 years and 56% at 10 years (Jenkins *et al.* 1999).

INDICATIONS FOR PITUITARY IRRADIATION

Over the past 40 years, the role of radiotherapy in the treatment of acromegaly has evolved through several phases of acceptance, side-by-side with advances in both neurosurgery and medical therapy, such as the development of somatostatin analogues, and in the near future possibly of GH receptor antagonists. Nowadays, the most common indication for pituitary irradiation is as second-line therapy in those patients whose GH levels remain elevated after pituitary surgery, or whose initially large tumours are incompletely resected by surgery. As a consequence of the relatively slow onset of action of irradiation, the residual GH hypersecretion requires suppression by concomitant medical therapy. However, regular withdrawal of such therapy is necessary to assess the effects of irradiation on underlying GH secretion. Of note is that the new long-acting somatostatin analogues may suppress GH secretion for up to 4 months after withdrawal. This means that the frequent assessment of irradiation efficacy can be problematical. It is our policy to switch such patients to short-acting subcutaneous somatostatin analogues for at least 3 months prior to reassessment with an additional 4–6 week drug-free interval to avoid any rebound hypersecretion of GH.

In patients for whom surgery is contraindicated for whatever reason, pituitary irradiation provides a safe and effective first-line therapy, although again medical therapy is likely to be required in the interim period until its effects become biochemically apparent.

Contraindications to pituitary irradiation are relatively few. The predominant concern relates to tumours with significant suprasella extension and actual or incipient optic nerve compression, as there is a risk, albeit probably small, that irradiation may result in oedema of the tumour with further compression. This can be prevented by prior surgery, with the aim being to debulk if not completely resect the adenoma. Conversely, a completely empty sella is also considered by some investigators to be a relative contraindication because of the possibility of irradiation-induced fibrosis drawing down the diaphragm and pulling on the chiasm.

SIDE EFFECTS OF IRRADIATION

Hypopituitarism

There is no doubt that hypopituitarism is the major disadvantage of pituitary irradiation. It has long been known that anterior pituitary deficiencies occur after radiotherapy in which the hypothalamo–pituitary axis is encompassed within the irradiation field. More recently, it has been shown that the deficiencies occur more as a result of hypothalamic dysfunction, and thus more focused irradiation on the pituitary that avoids the hypothalamic region may result in a reduced incidence of subsequent hypopituitarism, although long-term data regarding the effects of radiosurgery are required. The total dose prescribed and probably the dose per daily treatment fraction are the major factors that determine the risk and speed of onset of any radiation-induced hypopituitarism, although some evidence suggests that low-dose irradiation might be associated with a lower incidence of subsequent hypopituitarism (Littley *et al.* 1990). Regardless of this, the risk increases with time after therapy. Rises in PRL postradiotherapy also have their origins at the hypothalamic level, as may the observation of occasional early or accelerated puberty after pituitary radiation.

For as yet undetermined reasons, there are marked differences in the radiosensitivity of different hypothalamic and pituitary cell lineages; of benefit in the treatment of patients with acromegaly is that GH-secreting neurones are the most sensitive, followed by gonadotrophin-secreting ones, with those that secrete adrenocorticotrophin (ACTH) being less sensitive and thyroid-stimulating hormone (TSH) the least sensitive. Diabetes insipidus very rarely occurs. This is reflected in the incidence of radiation-induced hypopituitarism of the different axes. The overall incidence of hypopituitarism is greater the more abnormal is the pituitary function prior to radiotherapy (i.e. tumour or surgery related). Thus, 'percentage' statistics on the incidence of postradiotherapy hypopituitarism are not exact. Nevertheless, in the St Bartholomew's series of acromegalic patients, 25% required new endocrine replacement therapy by 5 years after radiotherapy and the need continued to rise in the next 5 years. Feek et al. (1984) reported that by 10 years postradiotherapy, 47% of patients were hypogonadal, 30% hypoadrenal and 16% hypothyroid. These incidences were 70%, 54% and 38%, respectively, when surgery preceded radiotherapy. The impact of prior surgery or of mass effects of the tumour itself on baseline pituitary function is illustrated by data from the UK National Acromegaly Study Group. By 10 years after irradiation, new deficiencies of gonadotrophins occurred in 29% of patients, while 8% developed new ACTH deficiency and none became hypothyroid.

Optic nerve damage

By observance of careful modern planning and dose prescription delivery, the risks to the normal optic chiasm should be extremely low. The pathological basis for radiation morbidity to the chiasm (via its vasa nervorum) is now better understood than 20 years ago. The major factors in the radiation prescription that contribute to the risk of optic chiasm damage are the total dose and the dose per fraction. While employing radiotherapy for pituitary adenoma in a dose range of 42–59 Gy in Boston between 1963 and1973, Harris and Levene (1976) found radiation-induced optic neuropathy in four out of 55 patients, but in none who received a daily dose per fraction <2.5 Gy. Aristazabal et al. (1977) reviewed 122 patients treated for pituitary adenoma with radiotherapy and found optic neuropathy in four cases – all four patients occurred in a subgroup of 26 patients who had received >46 Gy total dose and all four patients had received a daily dose >2.0 Gy per fraction. Other data support the conclusion that large daily dose fractions place the optic chiasm at greater risk. A long-term tumour-compressed chiasm with optic atrophy on fundoscopy prior to radiation therapy is also more vulnerable. In the past decade few instances of such damage have been recorded in the conventional radiotherapeutic literature, which testifies to the now general acceptance of these dose limitations for safety. In single arm series, using conventionally fractionated (2.0 Gy/day or less) radiotherapy, Brada et al. (1993) recorded two cases of late and otherwise unexplained visual deterioration in a series of 411 patients treated with doses up to 50 Gy (neither case resulted in blindness). Jones (1991) found no cases of late optic neuropathy in 332 patients treated to 45 Gy in 1.8 Gy daily fractions.

Carcinogenesis

It is probable that there may be a late risk of secondary carcinogenesis subsequent to pituitary irradiation, but whether it is as high as the often quoted 1–2% remains contentious (Jones 1991, Brada et al. 1992). In a long-term follow-up study of 334 patients treated for pituitary adenoma by radiotherapy, Brada et al. (1992) described the development of two gliomas, two meningiomas and one meningeal sarcoma, and concluded that the increased risk of developing second tumours following this procedure is 1.9% at 20 years. Tsang et al. (1993) observed the occurrence of four gliomas (two in the brainstem) in the long-term follow up of 367 irradiated pituitary adenoma patients and made similar conclusions. Jones (1991) reported the occurrence of one glioma, one peripheral neuroectodermal tumour and two cases of myelogenous leukaemia (one acute and one chronic) in the late follow up of 332 irradiated pituitary adenoma patients. However, he observed the occurrence of one glioma in a nonirradiated pituitary adenoma patient and warned of the use of background population statistic comparisons, advice our group has reiterated and that seems more pertinent in this age of research into GH tumour growth factors (Wass et al. 1992). Bliss et al. (1994) observed one malignant brain lymphoma in a patient who had also previously undergone chemotherapy for Hodgkin's disease, and one meningioma in the long-term follow up of 193 irradiated pituitary adenoma patients. If we total these four series, we find that, in the late follow up of 1226 irradiated pituitary adenoma patients, there have been seven gliomas, two benign meningiomas (although Tsang et al. (1993) might not have recorded benign tumours) and one malignant meningeal sarcoma/parasellar fibrosarcoma. When compared to background population incidences (e.g. three per 1000 for glioma), albeit with whatever shortcomings these data may have, it is clear that any excess risks are small. Furthermore, it is possible that patients with pituitary adenomas have a predisposition to other intracranial neoplasms per se, regardless of whether they have received irradiation. This would bias the observed prevalence of second malignancies in these patients with irradiation, given the absence of control groups of nonirradiated pituitary adenoma patients in most series.

Brain necrosis

There is a concern that localised radiotherapy to this area of brain might lead to more neuropsychological late changes than partial brain radiotherapy received by other brain sites or to the whole brain. However, although some workers have reported the occurrence of neurocognitive late morbidity following radiotherapy for pituitary adenoma, any changes were found to be unrelated to radiotherapy (Peace *et al.* 1997, 1998). It is reassuring that brain necrosis was not recorded in either of the two London group experiences of some 743 irradiated patients followed up long-term (Jones 1991, Brada *et al.* 1993). In another study, although there were more neuropsychological disturbances in pituitary adenoma patients than expected, it was uncertain whether these were related to previous radiotherapy. An English study found poor social adjustment, including mood disorders, to be related to radiotherapy, but as part of a multifactorial problem, to which surgery and hormonal imbalance also contributed (Peace *et al.* 1997, 1998). Further neuropsychological research is required before and after therapy in hypothalamopituitary tumour patients to clarify these issues.

STEREOTACTIC RADIOTHERAPY

Single, high-dose, stereotactically delivered radiation therapy ('radiosurgery') is a relatively less widely understood form of radiation therapy. Stereotactic technology allows precise target definition, thereby enabling the beam to be concentrated more specifically on the target (often only part of the fossa), which is mapped with millimetre precision via three-dimensional co-ordinates obtained with the patient immobilised in a stereotactic frame. The stereotactic technology thus allows a more highly 'focussed' (more properly, concentrated) dose, but also at the edge of the mapped target volume the dose 'falls off' very rapidly (i.e. faster than at the periphery of a conventionally treated target volume). Either high-energy photons (X-rays or gamma rays) or charged particles (protons or helium ions) can be administered in this way.

Currently, two photon stereotactic radiosurgical techniques are increasingly available. Both methods require the head to be fixed within a stereotactic mapping frame (*Fig. 6.4*). In the current design of the Swedish gamma unit (Gamma Knife, Electa Instruments AB, Linkoping, Sweden) there are 201 fixed cobalt-60 sources, each as a thin rod of 1 mm diameter, the long axis of which is oriented along the radius of a hemisphere (the helmet into which the patient's head fits). The centre point (or isocentre) of this hemisphere is the point at which the stereotactic co-ordinates of the mapped intracranial target, within the patient's head, are positioned. The 201 sources deliver their emissions through collimators with different apertures (4, 8, 14 or 18 mm diameter) – all positioned radially from the isocentre (*Fig. 6.5*).

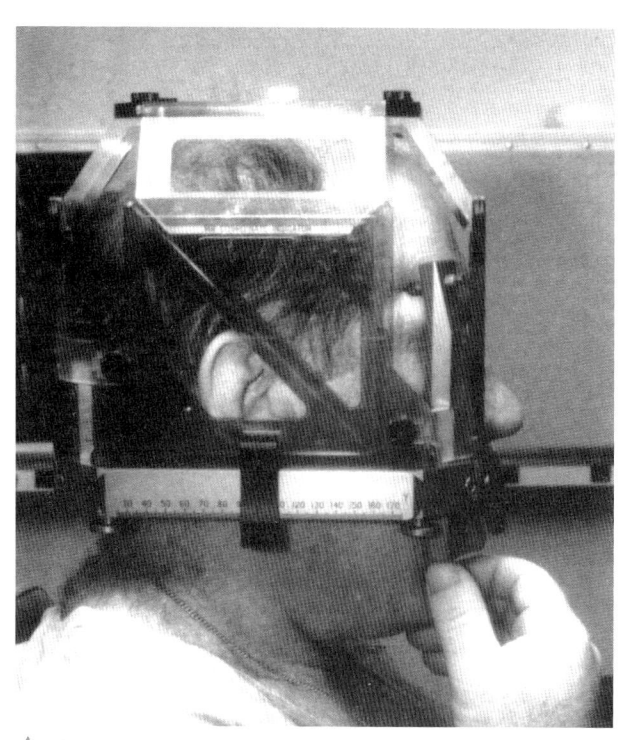

▲ **Figure 6.4** Patient in a stereotactic frame for gamma knife mapping.

The linear accelerator methodology again stereotactically maps the intracranial target by three-dimensional co-ordinates and places it at an isocentre, but this time it is an isocentre around which a single beam (emitting X-rays continuously) arcs. The planning software has acquired the name 'x-knife' (Radionics, MA, USA). Five 140° arcs are usually employed at our institution (but optimised for individuals); by the end of this a large dose has accumulated on the target, but the surrounding brain has received no more than a passing dose. Different collimator sizes allow different target sizes to be treated.

By combining multiple, differently isocentred treatments (where necessary) for each patient, the dose distribution may be conformed to irregular target volumes. Various fine adjustments allow a sharper than usual dose 'fall-off' at one border of the target volume, for both the gamma knife and x-knife units, and these may be particularly advantageous for tumours that approach the chiasm. This precise dose administration requires very accurate mapping of the target, with the tumour distribution delineated by modern MRI scanners linked to the planning equipment.

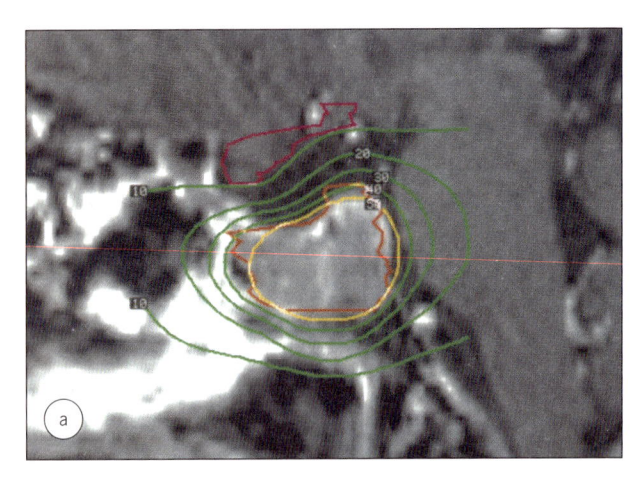

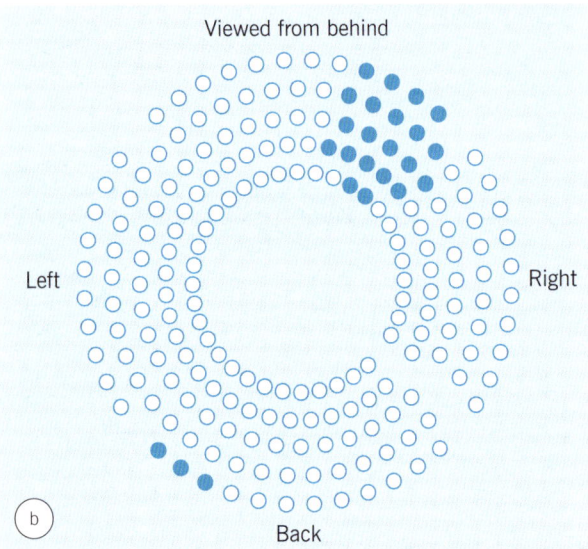

Figure 6.5 (a) Radiation isodosimetry achieved by gamma knife radiosurgery – target volume/pituitary adenoma (outlined in red) and optic chiasm (outlined in magenta) as imaged by sagittal MRI (T1-weighted). The isodosimetry of the gamma knife treatment is superimposed on the MRI (orange line represents 50% fall off, green lines represent further decreasing isodosimetry). Note that the isodoses fall faster on the rostral aspect of the target volume, adjacent to the optic chiasm. This is achieved by 'blocking' channels in the gamma knife treatment helmet facing the chiasm – a method of achieving an even steeper dose gradient on one aspect of the target; this is figuratively displayed in (b).

In several comparative studies, little difference was found between the basic single isocentre isodosimetry of the gamma knife versus x-knife photon methods, although recent publications (Plowman and Doughty 1999), which discuss more complex and commonly true-to-life situations, highlight some differences in the conformity indices and internal dose gradients that represent potentially important clinical differences. In our own dosimetric comparative study, we found a better gradient (i.e. faster 'fall off' of dose) could be achieved at the rostral border of the pituitary volume (i.e. that closest to the optic chiasm and hypothalamus) with the gamma unit than with linac technology – given the current technology to hand (Plowman and Doughty 1999).

Although radiosurgery has been used successfully for a number of years in the treatment of a variety of intracranial tumours, much of the initial data published on pituitary 'radiosurgery' have not been overly favourable. Kjellberg and Kliman (1979) published a large data set on proton beam therapy with generally good results. In a series of 234 unoperated acromegalic patients, there was a 70% decline in serum GH levels, which continued to the point of publication at up to 10 years, which was unquestionably a good and solid result.

In an early series on the efficacy of gamma knife radiosurgery in acromegaly, Thoren *et al.* (1991) reported that of 21 patients, seven received radiosurgery as primary therapy; of these two were cured and two improved. From Pittsburgh, Pollock *et al.* (1994) reported on the results of 35 patients treated with gamma knife technology, but of these only eight had acromegaly. Of these eight evaluable patients, serum GH was 'normalised' in three, decreased in three and increased in two. Two patients out of 35 developed complications in this series (one visual and one hypothalamic). The incidence of visual complications is perceived to be lower in the current series, in which a cap of 8 Gy to the chiasm is practised during single-fraction radiosurgery. Park *et al.* (1996) reported another series of 27 pituitary patients treated by the gamma knife. In three out of seven patients with acromegaly the GH serum levels returned to normal and a good response was seen in a fourth patient. In a Virginia (USA) series reported at a 1998 London symposium, Laws *et al.* (unpublished) found that 25% of 56 acromegalic patients had normal IGF-I levels by 20 months, with others continuing to improve.

Some more recent work appears to demonstrate better results for first-time cure with radiosurgery. Landolt *et al.* (1998) compared a nonrandomised series of 50 acromegalic patients treated with conventional radiotherapy (mean pretreatment GH level of 28 mU/l (14 μg/l) and follow-up period of 7.5 years), with 16 patients with acromegaly treated radiosurgically (mean presenting GH level of 18 mU/l (9 μg/l) and follow-up period of 1.4 years). They concluded that normalisation of GH occurs faster with the gamma knife (70% of the 16 patients achieved this by 18 months, whereas it took up to 7 years for the same percentage to achieve this following conventional radiotherapy). However, the radiosurgical follow-up period is short in comparison to the long-term conventional radiotherapy data, a problem with most radiosurgery results to date.

Our preliminary results at St Bartholomew's Hospital are in agreement with these findings (Swords et al. 2000). X-knife radiosurgery has been administered to 13 patients with acromegaly, all of whom had persistent GH hypersecretion despite previous surgery and conventional irradiation. Seven patients were also receiving somatostatin analogue therapy. Ten of the 13 patients had extension of the tumour outside the fossa into either the cavernous or sphenoid sinus. After an initial planning visit, all the patients received a single fraction of stereotactic irradiation at a mean dose of 10 Gy (range 8–15 Gy). To minimise any consequent tumour oedema we administered dexamethasone 4 mg 2 h before therapy and every 6 h afterwards for 36 h. After a median follow-up period of 18 months (range 3–48 months), all the patients showed a fall in serum GH and IGF-I levels. The mean GH declined from 21.8 mU/l (10.9 μg/l) to 9.5 mU/l (4.8 μg/l) with five patients having a level <5 mU/l (<2.5 μg/l). Similar impressive results were observed in the IGF-I levels, which declined from a mean of 632 ng/ml to 446 ng/ml, with six patients having a level within the age-matched normal range. MRI showed a reduction in tumour size in three patients. One patient reported a transient worsening of his headache following radiosurgery, although there were no other reported adverse effects. None of the patients has lost residual anterior pituitary function at their last assessment.

These results would seem to suggest that radiosurgery leads to fast and impressive falls in GH levels, even in previously irradiated patients, but that it is not appropriate for every case. A major concern regarding radiosurgery as primary radiation therapy for pituitary adenoma is that poor initial selection may prejudice later alternative therapy, as partial radiation tolerance will have been delivered. In addition, care needs to be taken if radiosurgery is advocated as primary therapy because the focussed irradiation will often result in a fibrotic gland, which makes any subsequent neurosurgical intervention technically difficult. Also, the lack of long-term recurrence data may be problematic. Clinicians must not be uncritical of the good initial falling hormone levels without knowing the long-term control data for this modality over conventionally fractionated, higher total-dose therapy; they must await follow-up data on radiosurgically treated patients of longer duration.

References

Aristizabal S, Caldwell WL & Avila J 1977 The relationship of time–dose fractionation factors to complications in the treatment of pituitary tumors by irradiation. *International Journal of Radiation Oncology, Biology, Physics* **2** 667–673.

Béclère A 1909 Le traitment médical des tumeurs hypophysaires du gigantisme et de l'acromégalie par la radio-thérapie. *Bulletins et Mémoires de la Société des Hôpitaux de Paris* **27** 274.

Biermasz NR, Van Dulken H & Roelfsema F 2000 Long-term follow-up results of postoperative radiotherapy in 36 patients with acromegaly. *Journal of Clinical Endocrinology and Metabolism* **85** 2476–2482.

Bliss P, Kerr GR & Gregor A 1994 Incidence of second brain tumours after pituitary irradiation in Edinburgh 1962–1990. *Clinical Oncology* **6** 361–363.

Brada M, Ford D, Ashley S et al. 1992 Risk of second brain tumour after conservative surgery and radiotherapy for pituitary adenoma. *British Medical Journal* **304** 1343–1346.

Brada M, Rajan B, Traish D et al. 1993 The long-term efficacy of conservative surgery and radiotherapy in the control of pituitary adenomas. *Clinical Endocrinology (Oxford)* **38** 571–578.

Ciccarelli EC, Orsello SH, Plowman PN et al. 1988 Prolonged lowering of growth hormone after radiotherapy in acromegalic patients followed over 15 years. In *Advances in Pituitary Adenoma Research, Advances in Biosciences*, Vol. 69, pp 260–272. Eds Landolt AM, Heitz PU, Zapf J, Girard J & Del Pozo E. Pergamon Press: Oxford.

Ciccarelli E, Corsello SM, Plowman PN et al. 1989 Long-term effects of radiotherapy for acromegaly on circulating prolactin. *Acta Endocrinologica (Copenhagen)* **121** 827–832.

Feek CM, McLelland J, Seth J et al. 1984 How effective is external pituitary irradiation for growth hormone-secreting pituitary tumors? *Clinical Endocrinology (Oxford)* **20** 401–408.

Harris JR & Levene MB 1976 Visual complications following irradiation for pituitary adenomas and craniopharyngiomas. *Radiology* **120** 167–171.

Jenkins PJ, Elliott EL, Carson MN & Bates PR 1999 Use of a National Database to explore the effects of pituitary irradiation on serum GH and IGF-I in acromegaly. *Journal of Endocrinology* **163** (Suppl.) OC4.

Jones A 1991 Radiation oncogenesis in relation to the treatment of pituitary tumours. *Clinical Endocrinology (Oxford)* **35** 379–397.

Kjellberg RN & Kliman B 1979 Life-time effectiveness: a system of therapy for pituitary adenomas, emphasising Bragg peak proton hypophysectomy. In *Recent Advances in the Diagnosis and Treatment of Pituitary Tumors*, pp 269–286. Ed Linfoot JA. New York: Raven Press.

Landolt AM, Haller D, Lomax N et al. 1998 Stereotactic radiosurgery for recurrent surgically treated acromegaly: comparison with fractionated radiotherapy. *Journal of Neurosurgery* **88** 1002–1008.

Littley MD, Shalet SM, Swindell R, Beardwell CG & Sutton ML 1990 Low-dose pituitary irradiation for acromegaly. *Clinical Endocrinology (Oxford)* **32** 261–270.

Park YG, Chang JW, Kim EY & Chung SS 1996 Gamma knife surgery in pituitary microadenomas. *Yonsei Medical Journal* **37** 165–173.

Peace KA, Orme SM, Sebastian JP *et al*. 1997 The effect of treatment variables on mood and social adjustment in adult patients with pituitary disease. *Clinical Endocrinology (Oxford)* **46** 445–450.

Peace KA, Orme SM, Padayatty SJ, Godfrey HP & Belchetz PE 1998 Cognitive dysfunction in patients with pituitary tumour who have been treated with transfrontal or transsphenoidal surgery or medication. *Clinical Endocrinology (Oxford)* **49** 391–396.

Plowman PN & Doughty D 1999 Stereotactic radiosurgery, X: clinical isodosimetry of gamma knife versus linear accelerator X-knife for pituitary and acoustic tumours. *Clinical Oncology* **11** 321–329.

Pollock BE, Kondziolka D, Lunsford LD & Flickinger JC 1994 Stereotactic radiosurgery for pituitary adenomas: imaging, visual and endocrine results. *Acta Neurochirurgia* **62**(Suppl.) 33–38.

Powell JS, Wardlaw SL, Post KD & Freda PU 2000 Outcome of radiotherapy for acromegaly using normalization of insulin-like growth factor I to define cure. *Journal of Clinical Endocrinology and Metabolism* **85** 2068–2071.

Sheline GE 1981 Pituitary tumours: radiation therapy. In *Clinical Endocrinology 1. The Pituitary*, pp 106–109. Eds Beardwell C & Robertson GL. London: Butterworths.

Swords FM, Allan CA, Sibtain A *et al*. 2000 Stereotactic multiple arc radiotherapy (SMART) as a salvage treatment for acromegaly. *Journal of Endocrinology* **164**(Suppl.) P57.

Thoren M, Rahn T, Guo WY & Werner S 1991 Stereotactic radiosurgery with the cobalt-60 gamma unit in the treatment of growth hormone-producing pituitary tumors. *Neurosurgery* **29** 663–668.

Tsang RW, Laperrier NJ, Simpson WJ, Brierley J, Panzarella T & Smyth HS 1993 Glioma arising after radiation therapy for pituitary adenoma. *Cancer* **72** 2227–2233.

Wass JAH, Besser GM, Grossman A, Plowman N & Meade TW 1992 Second brain tumour after treatment for pituitary adenoma. *British Medical Journal* **305** 253–254.

7

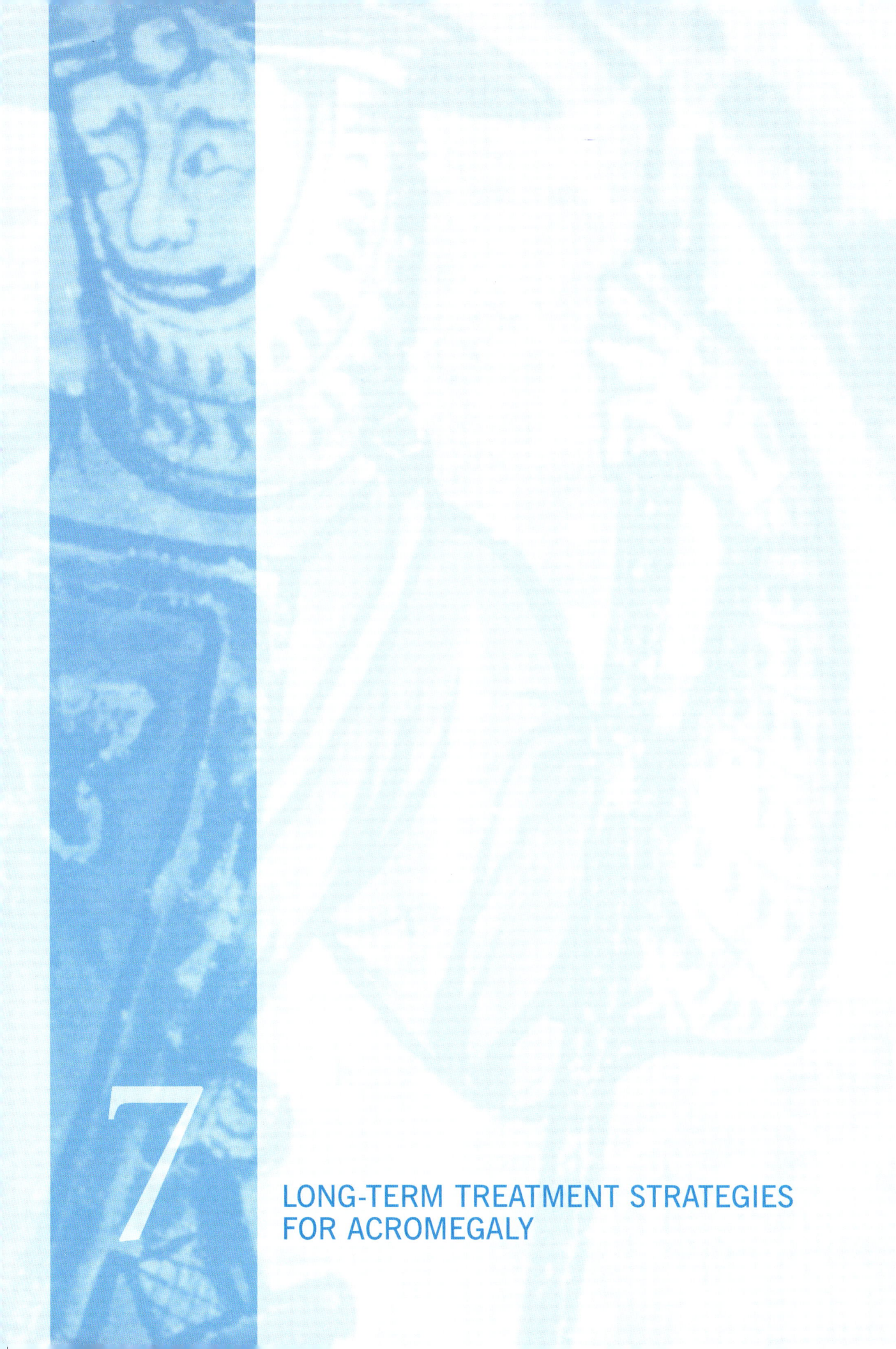

LONG-TERM TREATMENT STRATEGIES FOR ACROMEGALY

7 LONG-TERM TREATMENT STRATEGIES FOR ACROMEGALY

John Wass Department of Endocrinology, Radcliffe Infirmary, Oxford, UK
Steven Lamberts Department of Medicine, University Hospital of Rotterdam, Netherlands
Shlomo Melmed Cedars-Sinai Research Institute, Los Angeles, California, USA

INTRODUCTION

The objectives in the treatment of patients with acromegaly are described elsewhere (*see* Chapter 3). Treatment modalities include surgery using either the transsphenoidal or transcranial routes, drug treatment using somatostatin analogues, dopamine agonists or growth hormone (GH) receptor antagonists and radiotherapy – either external beam or gamma-knife radiotherapy.

Overall, microadenomas account for between 20 and 40% in individual series, and macroadenomas for the rest. It is, however, important to differentiate intrasellar macroadenomas, which have a different surgical outcome to extrasellar macroadenomas. This is discussed later.

In general, deciding the treatment strategy for an individual patient entails taking into account age and general health, presence of complications, severity of acromegaly and an assessment of the risks and/or benefits of each individual treatment. The size of the tumour and the GH levels have important bearings on the outcomes, but also the desire for fertility, particularly in the young, may have an important bearing on the individual treatment modality that is advised.

This chapter discusses each treatment modality for micro- and macroadenomas and then attempts to integrate a treatment strategy.

MICROADENOMAS

Surgery

Transsphenoidal surgery is currently the most frequently recommended primary treatment of microadenomas. In competent surgical hands between 80 and 90% of patients should have their GH levels rendered 'safe'. Both GH and insulin-like growth factor (IGF-I) levels fall rapidly and the attainment of safe GH levels is greater than that in drug treatment with somatostatin analogues (90% versus 60%). It has become clear, however, that only the best surgical results tend to be reported. An assessment of surgical outcome using data from individual centres contributing to the UK Acromegaly Database shows that the attainment of safe GH levels is less frequent than the best series in the literature – 80–90% versus 40–65% (Abosch *et al.* 1998, Swearingen *et al.* 1998, Ahmed *et al.* 1999, Bates *et al.* 2001). The cost of surgery relative to the cost of long-term therapy with drugs (e.g. somatostatin analogues) is low.

Postoperatively, the patient should be checked at 6 weeks. At this time GH levels and the individual reserves of the anterior pituitary hormones can be assessed. A postoperative magnetic resonance imaging (MRI) scan should be done at 6 months, because it usually takes at least this time for the appearances to settle postoperatively. This MRI acts as a baseline to assess later tumour regrowth. Provided radiotherapy is not administered the pituitary function usually remains unchanged after the first post-surgical check, and does not deteriorate futher.

A number of complications may arise from surgery, including loss of anterior pituitary function, diabetes insipidus, deterioration in visual fields, meningitis and haemorrhage. Overall these complications are not common (5%). Follow up is important, but recurrence (as distinct from persistence) of GH hypersecretion is fairly rare (7–10% at 5 years).

Medical treatment

The case has been made that in some patients primary medical treatment with octreotide should be considered (Freda *et al.* 1998). Reduction of GH is rapid, there is no loss of pituitary function and the long-term safety profiles of somatostatin analogues are reassuring. Particularly if the GH level is low pretreatment (20 mU/l (10 μg/l); Turner *et al.* 1999, Carson *et al.* 2001) the response rate in terms of normalisation of GH is around 80%. Overall though, taking pretreatment GH values of all patients into account, the response rate is about 60%. The cost of somatostatin is high, around £10,000 per year in the UK (equivalent to about 14,600 US$ or 15,900 euros per year), and there are side effects (see p. 56). This therapy needs to be monitored by measuring GH and IGF-I values, and ultrasound of the gallbladder is suggested, though symptomatic complications from gallstones are rare (<1%).

Dopamine agonists are effective much less frequently than somatostatin analogues, although they are easier to administer (being administrable orally). Less than 20% of patients obtain normal GH values (<5 mU/l (<2.5 µg/l)) and around 10% normal IGF-I values. The cost is clearly much less than that of somatostatin analogues. Few comparative studies have examined different dopamine agonists, but cabergoline seems more effective than bromocriptine, although these drugs have not been formally compared.

Pegvisomant, the GH receptor antagonist, renders IGF-I levels normal in >90% of patients with acromegaly. Currently, its long-term safety is unknown.

External pituitary radiotherapy

External pituitary radiotherapy should not be considered as primary therapy except in exceptional circumstances. The effects on GH and IGF-I levels are slow. At 10 years GH and IGF-I levels are <5 mU/l (<2.5 µg/l) in 50% of cases. There is an almost invariable decline in pituitary function such that at 10 years 70% of patients need replacement therapy, with sex steroids, thyroxine, hydrocortisone or a combination of these. The cost is low. Pulsatility of GH is effected such that GH deficiency can occur. Much less frequently, other side-effects can be seen; these include visual problems, particularly if the irradiation occurs with the pituitary tumour contiguous with the chiasm. Second malignancy can also occur in the field of radiotherapy and, although this is very infrequent indeed, such events occur at a rate of 2% in 20 years. It has been suggested that a psychological or memory deficit is consequent upon radiotherapy, but no reliable data have yet been published.

Gamma-knife radiotherapy is administered as a single dose and early reports suggest that the fall in GH levels is faster than that with ordinary external beam radiotherapy. Long-term follow-up studies have not as yet been published. Worldwide few machines are available so this treatment is not open to a large number of patients with acromegaly.

MACROADENOMAS

These may be either intra- or extrasellar. Extrasellar macroadenomas can involve the cavernous sinus or the sphenoid sinus. They may extend into the suprasellar space, where they may interfere with the optic pathways.

Surgery

With macroadenomas surgery is less effective than with microadenomas (Table 7.1). However, intrasellar macroadenomas have very similar surgical outcomes to those with microadenomas and between 70 and 80% of patients should have their GH levels rendered safe with effective surgery from an experienced surgeon. However, extrasellar macroadenomas have a considerably lower surgical success rate (see Chapter 4). Those in the cavernous sinus have 'safe' GH levels in <45% of cases postoperatively and those with large suprasellar extensions that compress the optic chiasm have safe postsurgical GH levels in <40% of cases.

Giant adenomas are virtually never cured using surgical treatment alone. Such adenomas often require transcranial surgery, usually following transsphenoidal surgery.

Transcranial surgery is necessary in a minority (3%) of patients with acromegaly.

Drugs

Octreotide has been suggested as a primary drug treatment for patients with macroadenomas. Particularly if the pretreatment GH level is very low, one might reasonably expect the attainment of safe GH levels in 60–80% of patients. As alluded to above it is clear that the frequency with which GH levels fall to normal is dependant on the pretreatment GH value. In the elderly with a small tumour, for example, and particularly those for whom surgery may be contraindicated by prior medical problems or in those who decline surgery, a case can be made for primary medical treatment using octreotide or lanreotide. In such patients some degree of tumour shrinkage can occur in 30–40% of patients, though the degree of tumour shrinkage is also modest, being >25% in only a quarter of patients treated.

We do not currently know whether the effect of somatostatin analogues is enhanced by lowering the GH level surgically. No studies have been carried out in which somatostatin analogues are given preoperatively and after unsuccessful surgery in the same

LONG-TERM TREATMENT STRATEGIES FOR ACROMEGALY

Table 7.1 Advantages and disadvantages of treatments for acromegaly.

ADVANTAGES AND DISADVANTAGES OF TREATMENTS FOR ACROMEGALY

Treatment		Advantages	Disadvantages
Surgery	Microadenomas	High cure rate, 80–90%	Loss of pituitary function, 12%
		Rapid GH/IGF-I reduction	Recurrence rate 7–10% at 5 years
		Low cost	Mortality (negligible)
	Macroadenomas	Rapid reduction of GH levels	<50% achieve safe GH values if extrasellar extension
Drugs	Somatostatin analogues	60% normal GH	Intramuscular injections
		Rapid GH reduction	Cost £10,000 (14,600 US$ or 15,900 euros) per year
		No loss of pituitary function	Side effects
		Long-term safety	
		Modest tumour shrinkage	
		Effect on GH suppression sustained	
	Dopamine agonists	Oral administration	GH normal in only 20%; high dose required
			Side effects
	GH receptor antagonists	IGF-I normal >90%	Long-term safety unknown
Radiotherapy	External beam	Low cost	Slow reduction in GH and IGF-I
			Control rate at 10 years, 50%
			Hypopituitarism in 70%
			Other side effects include visual loss in a small number of cases and possible second malignancy in the field of radiotherapy
			Possible effects on memory
	Gamma knife	Simple administration	Few machines available
			Long-term effects unclear

patients. Such prospective studies are of interest to establish whether the effect of somatostatin analogues is enhanced by surgical reduction in GH levels. Using somatostatin analogues as second-line (postsurgical) treatment only achieves normality in GH secretion in around 40% of cases (Newman et al. 1998).

Lastly, drugs may be used pre-surgery to decrease tumour size, but this has not been convincingly shown to improve surgical outcomes in terms of GH levels after surgery.

Radiotherapy

Radiotherapy is not advised as primary treatment for macroadenomas; some evidence indicates that it is particularly contraindicated in patients with compression of the optic chiasm who have not had surgical decompression because of the possibility of interfering with chiasmal blood flow. These patients may be more prone to visual complications from radiotherapy.

TREATMENT PARADIGMS

Surgery

In most patients surgery is the first-line treatment of choice (*Figure 7.1*). If surgery renders GH levels safe (GH nadir <2 mU/l (<1 μg/l) during oral glucose tolerance test (OGTT) and normal age- and sex-related IGF-I) following the postsurgical procedures described above, follow up should be yearly with annual measurements of GH and IGF-I to detect recurrence. Pituitary function will not change so that the regular assessments described do not need to include pituitary function once this has been adequately documented postoperatively.

TREATMENT PARADIGMS IN ACROMEGALY

Microadenoma → Surgery
- GH <5 mU/l (<2.5 μg/l) or GTT GH nadir <2 mU/l (<1 μg/l) IGF-I normal (90%)
- GH >5 mU/l (>2.5 μg/l) IGF-I high (10%)

Macroadenoma → Surgery
- GH >5 mU/l (>2.5 μg/l) IGF-I high (55%)
- GH <5 mU/l (<2.5 μg/l) or GTT GH nadir <2 mU/l (<1 μg/l) IGF-I normal (45%)

MEDICAL TREATMENT
Somatostatin analogues (60% normal IGF-I and GH <5 mU/L (<2.5 μg/l))
or
Dopamine agonists (10–20% GH <5 mU/l (<2.5 μg/l) IGF-I normal)
or
GH receptor antagonists (IGF-I normal >90%)

- GH <5 mU/l (<2.5 μg/l) IGF-I normal → Consider external beam radiotherapy
- GH >5 mU/l (>2.5 μg/l) IGF-I high → External beam radiotherapy

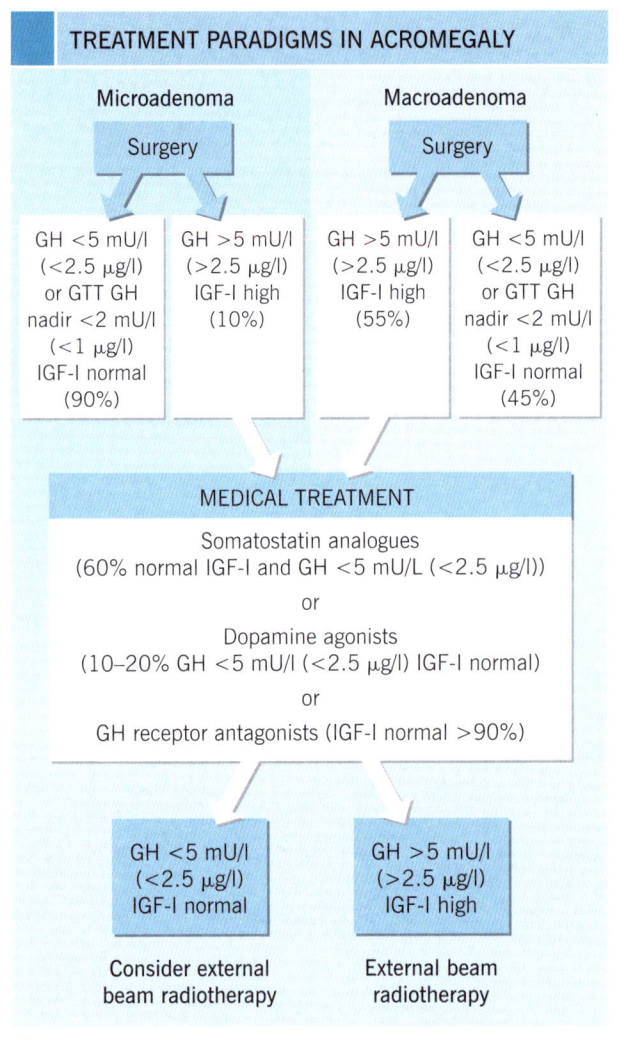

Figure 7.1 Treatment paradigms in acromegaly.

The second category of patients are those who are inadequately controlled (Giustina et al. 2000). These patients have a GH nadir of >2 mU/l (>1 μg/l) after OGTT, an elevated IGF-I, but no clinical activity. Occasionally GH and IGF-I data are discordant such that the GH response to oral glucose is normal but the IGF-I is elevated or indeed *vice versa*. There are no prospective controlled epidemiological data on whether these patients should be treated or not. In the decision-making process the metabolic and other effects, including those on the cardiovascular system, need to be taken into account. Thus, for example, a diabetic patient whose GH and IGF-I values are as above would be considered for treatment whereas a patient with no cardiovascular or metabolic consequences of acromegaly might simply be observed. Clearly, the risks and benefits of individual treatments have to be considered carefully in each patient that falls into this category.

The third group of patients who require further treatment following unsuccessful surgery are those in whom control is poor and who also have active acromegaly. Thus, in patients with a nadir GH level of >2 mU/l (>1 μg/l) after oral glucose and an elevated IGF-I there is a 3.5 fold increase in mortality, so treatment aimed at reducing GH levels is both desirable and necessary (Abosch et al. 1998).

In these circumstances medical treatment using octreotide or lanreotide, a dopamine agonist or GH receptor antagonists should be considered. If the response to medical treatment is inadequate, radiotherapy also needs to be considered. At this time it is also imperative to treat other co-morbidities associated with acromegaly, including hypertension, diabetes, heart disease, osteoarthritic complications of acromegaly and sleep apnoea. All of these have been associated with a higher mortality. For example, sleep apnoea has been associated with a higher frequency of myocardial infarction, hypertension and stroke.

Medical therapy

Octreotide or lanreotide should be considered currently as the first-line drugs in the medical treatment of acromegaly. An assessment using subcutaneous short-acting octreotide is made as to whether a GH response can be expected. If there is a satisfactory response this drug can be given long term and, cost considerations aside, this is perfectly acceptable because it is effective and its long-term safety is known.

A proportion of patients, however, do not respond to somatostatin analogues because their tumours do not bear somatostatin receptors, so in these circumstances it is wise to try dopamine agonists next (e.g. cabergoline). Although the response rate is lower, some evidence indicates a synergistic effect between dopamine agonists and somatostatin analogues, and a small proportion of patients who do not respond to somatostatin analogues respond to dopamine agonists. These drugs are tried next because of their comparative cost, which is low. If there is still inadequate GH suppression further surgery can be considered if there is residual tumour. It is usual, however, for a second surgery to be successful only when the first surgical attempt was made by a less experienced pituitary surgeon.

In patients for whom somatostatin analogues with or without cabergoline are not effective, the GH receptor antagonist pegvisomant may be used. Currently it is not licensed or available, but the studies carried out so far (Trainer et al. 2000) suggest that IGF-I levels are rendered normal in virtually all patients. The cost of this drug is currently unknown and there are no long-term safety data.

It is thus now possible to control by medical means the vast majority of patients who have active acromegaly following unsuccessful surgery. Of these, 50–60% are controllable with octreotide or lanreotide and the others may have their IGF-I values controlled by the use of pegvisomant.

Radiotherapy

External beam radiotherapy should be considered if there is no response to drugs in patients whose GH levels remain above normal after surgery. Recently, concerns about the use of radiotherapy have arisen. There are suggestions that cerebrovascular mortality increases after radiotherapy, but further epidemiological evidence is required. There are also suggestions that psychological sequelae to radiotherapy occur in terms of memory loss. Again, no satisfactory publications have confirmed or refuted this in patients who are properly replaced with all pituitary hormones, including GH. Furthermore, GH deficiency can be induced particularly with radiotherapy, and studies of GH pulsatility (Peacey et al. 1998) suggest that not only GH deficiency but also abnormalities of pulsation may occur. The onset of GH deficiency may be another cardiovascular risk factor that needs to be taken into account and occasionally the onset of GH deficiency (with all its attendant symptoms) after radiotherapy may require GH replacement therapy.

Finally, the administration of external beam radiotherapy requires regular monitoring of pituitary function on a yearly or biannual basis and invariably patients develop hypopituitarism which requires replacement therapy (70% require replacement therapy at 10 years).

Drugs to lower GH levels should be withdrawn at fairly regular annual or biannual intervals to assess the effects of radiotherapy on GH secretion. Clearly, they should not be continued when GH levels have been suppressed by radiotherapy.

CONCLUSIONS

We now have within our grasp the ability to reduce GH levels to safe values in all but the smallest minority of patients. Mostly this is achieved with surgery and somatostatin analogues. Pegvisomant has the potential to normalise IGF-I values in the vast majority of patients.

All patients with low GH values do well with all modalities of treatment, including surgery, somatostatin analogues and radiotherapy. A converse of this is that patients with high GH values and/or large pituitary tumours respond poorly to all modalities of treatment, including surgery, medical treatment and radiotherapy.

In particular, in patients with acromegaly who are young and especially prone to harbour large pituitary tumours, the judicious use of all modalities of treatment is necessary, either sequentially or in combination.

References

Abosch A, Tyrrell JB, Lambrown KR, Hannegan LT, Applebury CB & Wilson CB 1998 Transsphenoidal microsurgery for growth hormone secreting pituitary adenomas: initial outcome and long-term results. *Journal of Clinical Endocrinology and Metabolism* **83** 3411–3418.

Ahmed S, Elsheikh M, Stratton IM, Page RCL, Adams CBT & Wass JAH 1999 Outcome of transsphenoidal surgery for acromegaly and its relationship to surgical experience. *Clinical Endocrinology* **50** 561–567.

Bates P, Carson MN & Wass JAH 2001 Surgical outcomes for acromegaly vary widely: a report on behalf of the UK National Pituitary Database. To be presented at ENDO 2001 (American Endocrine Society), Denver.

Carson MN, Bates P & Wass JAH 2001 Somatostatin analog therapy for acromegaly in clinical practice: a report on behalf of the UK National Pituitary Database. To be presented at ENDO 2001 (American Endocrine Society), Denver.

Freda PU, Post KD, Powell JS & Wardlaw SL 1998 Evaluation of disease status with sensitive measures of growth hormone secretion in 60 postoperative patients with acromegaly. *Journal of Clinical Endocrinology and Metabolism* **83** 3808–3816.

Giustina A, Barkan A, Casanueva FF et al. 2000 Criteria for cure of acromegaly: a consensus statement. *Journal of Clinical Endocrinology and Metabolism* **85** 526–529.

Newman CB, Melmed S, George A et al. 1998 Octreotide as primary therapy for acromegaly. *Journal of Clinical Endocrinology and Metabolism* **83** 3034–3040.

Peacey SR, Toogood AA & Shalet SM 1998 Hypothalamic dysfunction in 'cured' acromegaly is treatment modality dependent. *Journal of Clinical Endocrinology and Metabolism* **83** 1682–1686.

Swearingen B, Barker FG, Katznelson L et al. 1998 Long-term mortality after transsphenoidal surgery and adjunctive therapy for acromegaly. *Journal of Clinical Endocrinology and Metabolism* **83** 3419–3426.

Trainer PJ, Drake WM, Katznelson L et al. 2000 Treatment of acromegaly with the growth hormone receptor antagonist pegvisomant. *New England Journal of Medicine* **342** 1171–1177.

Turner HE, Vadivale A, Keenan J & Wass JAH 1999 A comparison of lanreotide and octreotide LAR for treatment of acromegaly. *Clinical Endocrinology (Oxford)* **51** 275–280.

8

FUTURE AREAS OF RESEARCH
IN ACROMEGALY

8 FUTURE AREAS OF RESEARCH IN ACROMEGALY

John Wass Department of Endocrinology, Radcliffe Infirmary, Oxford, UK
Shlomo Melmed Cedars-Sinai Research Institute, Los Angeles, California, USA
Helen E Turner Department of Endocrinology, Radcliffe Infirmary, Oxford, UK

The successful treatment of acromegaly remains a therapeutic challenge. Despite advances in achieving control of growth hormone (GH) hypersecretion and tumour mass effects, it is clear that the total 'cure' of these patients, with normalised morbidity and mortality outcomes, is still difficult to achieve.

THE GENETIC BASIS OF THE PITUITARY TUMOUR

Currently, little is known about what controls pituitary tumour activity. We know that activating and inactivating genes are involved, particularly in some aggressive tumours, and that GS alpha mutations are seen in a proportion of Caucasian tumours secreting GH. Usually, these tumours are non-hereditary and have a lower blood vascularity than the normal pituitary, though it is not yet certain that the transforming gene for the human pituitary tumour induces angiogenesis (Ishikawa *et al.*, 2001). We do not know why there are differences between the young and the old in terms of tumour size or why tumours tend to be so much larger in younger patients. Although several growth factors have been implicated in dysregulated pituitary cell growth, little is known of their mechanistic and initiating actions. These growth factors include transforming growth factor, epidermal growth factor and vascular endothelial growth factor.

GROWTH HORMONE AND ASSAYS

One of the most significant problems that has bedevilled the acromegaly literature is that the values in GH assays have changed over the years; large numbers of contributions to the literature have used different, often imprecise, assays with poorly standardised controls and different applied criteria for the assessment of disease control or 'cure'.

Sensitivity of GH assays continues to improve. Currently, immunoradiometric assays are used widely, but it is likely that even more sensitive enzyme-linked immunoabsorbent assays will be used in the future. These will all have different normal ranges, and newly defined levels of GH will be deemed safe and associated with cure.

Ideally, these assays should be rigorously standardised, which might be possible in the UK, for example. This would offer the potential of data that are comparable between centres in a disease that requires large numbers of patients (unattainable in a single centre) to provide reliable and valid epidemiological data.

EPIDEMIOLOGICAL DATA

Using databases that are already operative in the UK and USA, we will be able to provide exciting new data on epidemiological aspects of acromegaly which have hitherto proved elusive. Currently, very little reliable evidence supports insulin-like growth factor-I (IGF-I) as the clinically relevant tumour marker rather than GH. We require prospective data that link IGF-I levels to mortality outcome. Is the sex- and gender-related IGF-I concentration alone, if normalised, enough to normalise mortality and morbidity in acromegaly?

These databases will also provide epidemiological data on patients who have evidence of mild biochemical acromegaly, but few or no clinical symptoms. We also need to know about mortality and morbidity in subcategories of patients with acromegaly; for example, in those administered radiotherapy alone, surgery alone or medical treatment with somatostatin (SST) analogues alone. There is a suggestion, for example, that radiotherapy increases the subsequent incidence of cardiovascular and cerebrovascular mortality (Tomlinson *et al.*, 2001). Furthermore, these databases will enable us to examine the long-term effects of GH deficiency that result from treatment to reduce GH levels. Does this have an adverse effect on life expectancy? Last, but by no means least, we should be able to obtain reliable epidemiological data on whether cancer incidence (including breast and colon cancer) is more common in patients with controlled and uncontrolled acromegaly.

SURGERY

Surgery (usually via the transsphenoidal route) remains the primary therapeutic strategy in patients with acromegaly, especially those with small, discrete intrasellar adenomas. Surgical experience is important and close collaboration with colleagues in endocrinology, imaging, radiotherapy and pathology is essential. New surgical techniques require evaluation as to whether they improve patient outcome. These include endoscopy, intraoperative hormone assays and magnetic resonance imaging examinations. It is hoped, for example, that endoscopic surgery will enable more efficient access to tumour tissue situated in the cavernous sinuses, as it is these commonly encountered tumours that tend to have poorer surgical and endocrine outcomes than those tumours confined to the pituitary fossa itself.

We need to develop standards for reporting surgical complications so that different surgeons and different centres can be compared more rigorously than was hitherto possible.

There are early indications that, in selected patients, pre-operative treatment with octreotide may be useful if they have serious medical complications of acromegaly (Colao et al., 1997). We do not yet have enough prospective data to compare GH levels pre- and postoperatively and so be able to say conclusively whether surgery to debulk a tumour is actually worthwhile if presurgical medical treatment has already produced a marked reduction in the GH level.

IMAGING

Novel imaging technology and three-dimensional techniques should further improve tumour visualisation, especially for distinguishing persistent or recurrent tumour progression from normal tissue or from postoperative changes.

MEDICAL TREATMENT

Medical treatment of acromegaly has progressed enormously since the 1970s and 1980s, with the advent first of dopamine agonists, then of SST analogues (including long-acting depot preparations of these compounds) and, recently, of GH receptor antagonists. We need to know more about the effects of selective analogues, particularly those specific for SST receptor subtype 2 and possibly analogous combinations. These subtype-selective analogues are in development. We need to know more about primary medical treatment of acromegaly which, cost apart, will probably control tumour growth long term in responsive patients. In addition, it may be particularly helpful in patients with initially low GH levels or in those, such as the elderly, with serious medical complications of acromegaly, and it may be less dangerous than surgery. New methods of SST analogue delivery are being developed and, for example, studies of lanreotide autogel are providing promising results that suggest its drug efficacy lasts for at least 4 weeks, suppressing GH in patients with persistent acromegaly.

We need to know the long-term safety profile of pegvisomant and its effect on pituitary tumour size (van der Lely et al., 2001). As alluded to above few data are available on the relationship between IGF-I levels and mortality and morbidity, and measuring IGF-I is currently the only means available to monitor pegvisomant therapy. More data are required here too.

RADIOTHERAPY

Conventional radiotherapy, which has been around for many years, is on the whole safe. We know the conventional dose used renders both GH and IGF-I normal in around 50% of patients after 10 years, but the effects are slow and hypopituitarism is common. In terms of tumour control it is unlikely that using a lower dose, which may be associated with a lower frequency of hypopituitarism, will be as effective. We need more data on cerebrovascular mortality after radiotherapy (Tomlinson et al., 2001) and on secondary malignancy arising in the field of the radiotherapy. More studies are required on the neuropsychological effects of radiotherapy for pituitary tumours and we need to be vigilant for the development of visual problems. When these do occur, we need to analyse the reasons in order to substantiate or refute the current prejudice that elderly hypertensive patients, in whom the tumour abuts the optic chiasm at the time of the radiotherapy, are more prone to this complication than are other patients.

In early assessments, gamma knife radiotherapy (radiosurgery) appears to reduce GH more quickly than conventional external beam radiotherapy. Formal comparisons can and should be made prospectively between gamma knife radiosurgery and conventional radiotherapy, perhaps from different centres, using tumours of comparable size as a baseline. This will provide data on the complication rates of hypopituitarism and, of course, on comparative rates of GH reduction, as well as on rates of tumour control.

OTHER DISEASES

Patients with acromegaly have enabled progress to be made in the study of other diseases seen in acromegaly, such as gallstones and colonic polyps. Gallstones that develop on SST therapy are related to changes in intestinal transit, bacterial flora and resultant alterations in bile, as well as to inhibition of gall bladder motility induced by cholecystokinin suppression.

Colonic cancer and colonic polyp prevalence may or may not be increased in acromegaly. Currently, the screening policy is arbitrarily defined as a colonoscopy every 3–5 years, but we need evidence to establish a firmer scientific basis for this. Certainly, insight into the development of colonic polyps and colonic cancer has been gained and we know, for example, that IGF-I receptors are expressed on colonic polyps and that patients with persistently active acromegaly are more likely to redevelop these than those in whom this is not the case (Jenkins *et al.*, 2000).

REPORTING TO SIMILAR CRITERIA

The recent development of criteria for the definition of safe GH levels or 'cure' of acromegaly is very important if we are to obtain good epidemiological data and compare outcomes in different centres (Giustina *et al.*, 2000). It is important that the endocrinology community recognise these new criteria and that they are used widely by authors and referees to ensure, as far as possible, a degree of consistency and uniformity within the acromegaly literature, which has hitherto been lacking.

CONCLUSIONS

Exciting times lie ahead in the study of this fascinating disease. We now have it within our grasp to control the vast majority of patients in terms both of tumour mass and of GH and IGF-I hypersecretion. Epidemiological data will hopefully continue to confirm that such control has a major effect not only on the mortality, but also on the morbidity of the disease. Ultimately, our patients will benefit from these fundamental advances in diagnosis and therapy.

References

Colao A, Ferone D, Cappabianca P *et al*. 1997 Effect of octreotide pre-treatment on surgical outcome and acromegaly. *Journal of Clinical Endocrinology and Metabolism* **82** 3308–3314.

Giustina A, Barkan A, Casanueva FF *et al*. 2000 Criteria for cure of acromegaly: a consensus statement. *Journal of Clinical Endocrinology and Metabolism* **85** 526–529.

Ishikawa H, Heaney AP, Yu R, Horwitz GA & Melmed S 2001 Human pituitary tumour-transforming gene induces angiogenesis. *Journal of Clinical Endocrinology and Metabolism* **86** 867–874.

Jenkins PJ, Frajese V, Jones A-M C *et al*. 2000 Insulin-like growth factor I and the development of colorectal neoplasia in acromegaly. *Journal of Clinical Endocrinology and Metabolism* **85** 3218–3221.

Tomlinson JW, Holden N, Hills RK *et al*. 2001 Association between premature mortality and hypopituitarism. *The Lancet* **357** 425–431.

van der Lely AJ, Muller AF, Janssen JA *et al*. 2001 Control of tumour size and disease activity during co-treatment with octreotide and the growth hormone receptor antagonist pegvisomant in an acromegalic patient. *Journal of Clinical Endocrinology and Metabolism* **86** 478–481.

INDEX

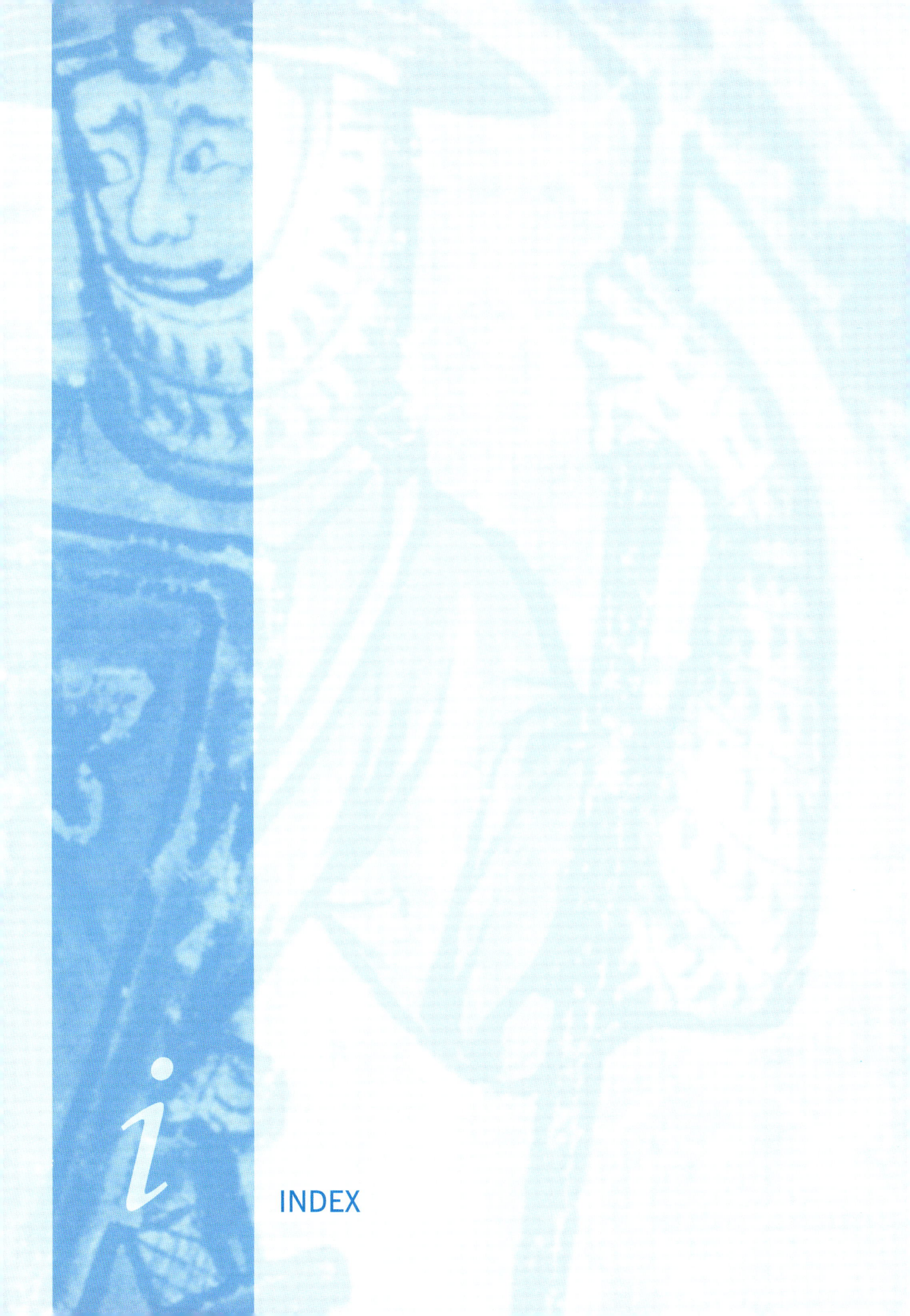

INDEX

A
acidophil stem-cell adenoma 22
acromegaly, origin of term 6
adrenocorticotrophic hormone (ACTH) 27
    deficiency 23, 34, 72
    tumours secreting 51–2
alpha-adrenergic antagonists 11
arrhythmias 24
arthropathy 25, 32

B
Bates, Captain 3, 4
Béclère, A 7, 8, 67
Bigfoot 4
Bill, Pecos 4
biochemical tests 25–6
bone disorders 25, 27
brain necrosis, radiation-induced 72–3
breast cancer 24, 52
bromocriptine 11, 56, 57–8
    stimulation test 26
Byrne, Charles 3, 4–5

C
cabergoline 57–8
calcium, increased levels 25, 27, 33
cAMP-response element binding protein (CREB) 21
cancer, see malignant disease
carbohydrate intolerance 24, 27, 33
carcinoid tumours 52
cardiac disease 24
    effects of treatment 32, 56
    investigations 27
cardiovascular disease 19, 24
Carney syndrome 20
carpal tunnel syndrome 25, 32
cause of acromegaly, determination 26–7
cavernous sinus, adenomas invading 42, 43, 80, 88
cerebrovascular disease 19, 83, 88
Chang Nu Sing 3, 4, 5
chlorpromazine 11
cholesterol, total serum 60
clinical features of acromegaly 22–5
    assessment 27
    reversibility 32
colonic polyps/cancer 24, 32, 89
colonoscopic screening 24, 89
complications of acromegaly, see clinical features of acromegaly
Cumhaill, Fionn mac 4
cure of acromegaly
    definitions 31, 35–6
        currently accepted 35–6, 51, 69
        historical 7–8
        importance of using 89
        surgical studies 41, 42, 44–5
        rates 32–3
    medical therapy 32, 33, 54–5, 58
    radiotherapy 32, 33, 69–70
    surgery 32, 33, 43–5
Cushing, Harvey 5, 6, 8, 9–10
Cushing's disease 34, 51
cutis verticis gyrata 23
cyclin-dependent kinase (CDK) inhibitors 21

D
dexamethasone 75
diabetes insipidus 71
diabetes mellitus 24, 33
diabetic nephropathy 59
diagnosis of acromegaly 25–7
    see also cure of acromegaly
disturbance, patient 34
dopamine 11
dopamine agonists 34, 56–8, 80
    efficacy 32, 33–4
    history 11
    role in therapy 63, 81, 82
    side effects 34–5, 58
dopaminergic tests 26
dose, radiation 68, 70
Dott, Norman 10
drug treatment, see medical therapy

E

electrocardiogram (ECG) 24
endocrine dysfunction 25
endoscope-assisted microsurgery 46, 88
epidemiological data 87–8
epidemiology of acromegaly 19
Evans, William 3, 4

F

facial features 23
familial acromegaly 20
fasting 58
fractionation, radiation dose 68

G

Galen (of Pergamum) 6
gallstones 56, 80, 89
gamma knife radiosurgery 73–5, 80
    efficacy 32, 33
    research needs 88–9
    role in therapy 81
GH, *see* growth hormone
giants 3–5
    biblical 3, 4
    historical 3, 4–5
    legendary 3–4
Giant's Causeway 4
gigantism 19
glucose tolerance
    effects of treatment 33, 56
    impaired 24
    test, *see* oral glucose tolerance test
Gogmagog 4
goitre 24, 25
Goliath 3, 4
gonadotrophins 27
    deficiency 23, 34, 72
G protein, stimulatory (gsp), mutations 21, 87
Greek mythology 3–4
growth factors 21, 87
growth hormone (GH)
    antibodies 60
    assays 36, 87
    clearance 60
    deficiency 83, 87
    ectopic hypersecretion 20
    historical studies 7
    hypersecretion 19–20, 22
    serum
        day curve 26
        defining cure, *see* cure of acromegaly, definitions

growth hormone (*cont.*)
    serum (*cont.*)
        dopamine agonist-treated patients 56, 57–8
        mortality and 19
        normalisation 32–3
        pegvisomant-treated patients 60–1
        pre-treatment 8, 45, 70, 79–80
        radiation-treated patients 68–70, 74–5
        random or basal 25, 35
        safe 31, 89
        somatostatin analogue-treated patients 54–5
    units 19
    urinary 26
growth hormone receptor antagonists 58–61, 81
    efficacy 32, 33, 59
    serum GH and 60–1
    side effects 59–60
    tumour size effects 61
    see also pegvisomant
growth hormone-releasing hormone (GHRH) 7
    in GH-secreting adenoma pathogenesis 21
    hypersecretion 20, 22
    serum 26
    stimulation test 26
Guiot, Gerard 10

H

hair loss 35, 56
Hardy, Jules 10
headache 23, 53
hereditary syndromes, associated 20
Hirsch, Oskar 8, 10
histopathology of acromegaly 22
history of acromegaly 3–15
Horsley, Sir Victor 8, 9
hypercalciuria 25, 27, 33
hyperprolactinaemia 20, 23
hypertension 24, 27, 32
hyperthyroidism 22, 25
hypopituitarism
    in acromegaly 23
    complicating radiotherapy 71–2, 80, 83
    complicating therapy 32, 34
hypothalamus
    in acromegaly pathogenesis 21
    regulation of GH secretion 7
hypothyroidism (TSH deficiency) 23, 34, 72

I

IGF-I, *see* insulin-like growth factor-I
imaging 26–7, 88
    see also magnetic resonance imaging

inferior petrosal sinus sampling (IPSS) 26
insulin-like growth factor-I (IGF-I)
   history 7
   inhibition of GH release 60
   malignancy and 24
   pathogenic role 19–20
   serum
      defining cure 36, 41, 51
      in diagnosis 25–6
      dopamine agonist-treated patients 56, 57–8
      epidemiological data needs 87
      mortality and 19
      normalisation 32, 33
      pegvisomant-treated patients 59
      radiation-treated patients 70–1, 75
insulin-like growth factor binding protein 1 (IGFBP1) 53
insulin-like growth factor binding protein 3 (IGFBP3) 26
insulin resistance 24, 59
investigations 25–7
islet cell tumours 52

J

joint disorders 25, 32

L

lanreotide 52
   autogel 53, 62, 88
   efficacy 33, 53–5
   slow-release (lanreotide-SR) 53, 62
L-dopa 11
life expectancy 35, 36
liver function tests, pegvisomant and 60, 62
loss of heterozygosity (LOH) 21

M

McCune–Albright syndrome 20
macroadenomas 22, 80–1
   extrasellar 43, 44, 45, 80
   intrasellar (IS) 43–4, 80
   outcome of surgery 32, 33, 43–4, 45
   treatment strategies 80–1, 82
macroglossia 23
magnetic resonance imaging (MRI) 26, 27
   intraoperative 47
   postoperative 79
   radiotherapy planning 67, 68
malignant disease (cancer)
   future data needs 87–8
   risk in acromegaly 19, 24–5, 27
   secondary to radiotherapy 35, 72, 88
mammosomatotroph tumours 22

Marie, Pierre 6
medical therapy 51–64, 79–81
   approach 63
   efficacy 32, 33–4, 54–5, 58
   future prospects 88
   history 8, 11
   modalities compared 61–2
   patient disturbance 34
   pros and cons 81
   in radiation-treated patients 71
   role 81, 82–3
   side effects 34–5
   see also dopamine agonists; growth hormone receptor
      antagonists; somatostatin analogues
medroxyprogesterone 11
menstrual disturbances 23
microadenomas 22
   outcome of surgery 32, 33, 43–4, 45
   treatment strategies 79–80, 81, 82
Miller, Maximilian Christopher 3, 4
mortality
   acromegaly 19
   complicating therapy 32, 35
   future data needs 87
   surgery 43
MRI, see magnetic resonance imaging
multiple endocrine neoplasia type 1 (MEN 1) 20, 25
myopathy, proximal 25

N

nasal approach, direct 46–7
neuromuscular disorders 25
neuronavigation 47
neuropsychological sequelae, radiotherapy 72–3, 83, 88
Norse mythology 4

O

O'Brien, Patrick 3, 4
octreotide 52, 79–80
   efficacy 33, 53–5
   inhibition of GH release 60
   long-acting repeatable (octreotide-LAR) 34, 53, 62
   somatostatin receptor subtypes and 52–3
   synergism with pegvisomant 61
oestrogen therapy 11, 58
oncogenes 21
optic nerve, radiation-induced damage 72
oral glucose tolerance test (OGTT)
   in definition of cure 31, 35–6, 41
   in diagnosis of acromegaly 25
osteoarthritis 25, 32
osteopenia 25

P

pathogenesis
    acromegaly 7, 19–21
    pituitary adenomas 20–1
Paul, F T 8, 9
Payne, Antony 3, 4
pegvisomant 34, 58–61, 80
    antibodies 60
    efficacy 32, 33, 34, 59
    mode of action 58–9
    research needs 88
    role in therapy 61–2, 63, 82–3
    serum GH levels and 60–1
    side effects 35, 59–60
    tumour size effects 61
phentolamine 11
pituitary
    apoplexy 23
    function tests 27
    historical aspects 6
    irradiation, *see* radiotherapy
pituitary adenomas 20
    genetic basis 21, 87
    giant, outcome of surgery 43, 44, 45, 80
    histopathology 22
    invasive 22
        outcome of surgery 43, 44, 45
        surgical treatment 42, 43
    mass/size
        direct effects 23
        efficacy of radiotherapy and 70
        reduction 33–4, 54, 61, 62
    pathogenesis 20–1
    recurrence 32, 34
    somatostatin receptors (SSTR) 21, 51–2
    surgery, *see* surgery
    see also macroadenomas; microadenomas
pituitary carcinoma 20, 22, 45
pituitary tumour transforming gene (PTTG) 21
Potsdam Giants 3, 4
prolactin (PRL)
    effects of cabergoline 57
    hypersecretion 20, 22, 23
    radiotherapy and 70
    serum 27
    somatostatin analogues and 53
prosopectasia 5
prostate cancer 24
protein 53 (p53) mutations 21

Q

quality of life (QoL), medical therapy and 53
quinagolide 56–7, 58

R

radiation dose 68, 70
radiography, plain 26
radiosurgery 67, 68, 73–5
    gamma knife, *see* gamma knife radiosurgery
    x-knife 73–4, 75
radiotherapy 67–76
    aims 32
    external beam 80, 81, 83
        complications 34, 35, 71–3, 80
        efficacy 32, 33, 34, 68–71
        history 7–8
        patient disturbance 34
    future prospects 87, 88–9
    indications 71, 82
    interstitial 8–9
    role 81, 83
    stereotactic 73–5
    theoretical aspects 67–8
    see also radiosurgery
remission of acromegaly, *see* cure of acromegaly
renal stones 25, 33
research, future needs 87–9
respiratory disease 19, 24, 27
retinoblastoma (Rb) gene 21
reversibility of somatic changes 32

S

Sasquatch 4
Schloffer, Herman 8, 9
scintigraphy, somatostatin receptor 27
serotonin antagonists 11
Sing, Chang Nu 3, 4, 5
skin changes 23–4
sleep apnoea 24, 82
sodium retention 24, 32
soft-tissue changes 23–4, 32
somatomedins 7
somatostatin 7, 51
    in pituitary adenoma pathogenesis 21
    therapy 11, 80
somatostatin analogues 51–6, 79–81
    adverse effects 34, 35, 56
    development 52
    efficacy 32, 33, 53–5
    long-acting formulations 53
    new 53
    postsurgical therapy 80–1
    preoperative therapy 55–6, 88
    in radiation-treated patients 71
    receptor subtypes and 52–3
    role in therapy 61–2, 63, 81, 82
    see also lanreotide; octreotide

somatostatin receptors (SSTR) 51–2
   in pituitary adenomas 21, 51–2
   scintigraphy 27
   subtype 2 selective analogues 53, 88
   subtype 5 selective analogues 53
   subtypes 52–3
somatotroph
   adenomas 22
   hyperplasia 20, 22
somatotrophinoma 20
somatotrophin release-inhibiting factor (SRIF) 7
somatotroph–lactotroph adenomas, mixed 22
sphenoid sinus, adenomas invading 43, 80
stereotactic ablation procedures 11–12
stereotactic radiotherapy, see radiosurgery
surgery 41–7
   case series (1982–2000) 41–4
      endocrinological evaluation 41
      procedures 42
      results 43–4
   complications 34, 43, 79
   efficacy 32, 33, 43–5
   future prospects 88
   goals 44
   history 8, 9–12
   mortality 43
   new techniques 46–7, 88
   patient disturbance 34
   radiotherapy after 70
   repeat 44, 46
   role 81–2
   somatostatin analogue pretreatment 55–6, 88
   unsuccessful 82, 83
Swan, Anna 3, 4
sweating 23, 32
symptoms of acromegaly 22–5
   relief of 31–2, 53

T

thyroid cancer 24
thyroid-stimulating hormone (TSH) 27
   deficiency 23, 34, 72
   hypersecretion 22, 25

thyrotoxicosis 22, 25
thyrotrophin-releasing hormone (TRH) test 26
transcranial surgery 80
   history 8, 10
   procedure 42
   results 44
transsphenoidal surgery 34, 79
   history 8, 9–11
   new techniques 46, 88
   procedure 42
   results 43–4
treatment of acromegaly
   aims 31–5
   efficacy 31–4
   future prospects 87–9
   history 7–12
   paradigms 81–3
   patient disturbance 34
   pros and cons of specific 81
   side effects 34–5
   strategies 79–83
   see also medical therapy; radiotherapy; surgery
TSH, see thyroid-stimulating hormone
tumour suppressor genes 21

V

vapreotide 52
Verga, Andrea 5
vision testing 26–7
visual impairment
   in acromegaly 23
   treatment-associated 35, 72, 74
voice, changes in 24

X

x-knife radiosurgery 73–4, 75

Y

Yeti 4
yttrium-90 (^{90}Y), interstitial therapy 8–9